LEAN FOR LONG-TERM CARE AND AGING SERVICES

Lean for Long-term Care and Aging Services. Copyright © 2014 by Sean Carey.

All rights reserved.

Second Edition
Version 1.1

LEAN FOR LONG-TERM CARE AND AGING SERVICES

A PRACTICAL GUIDE FOR DRIVING IMPROVEMENT, ENGAGEMENT, AND RESIDENT-CENTERED SERVICE

Sean Carey

TABLE OF CONTENTS

Introduction v
Lean Philosophy 2
    Lean Philosophy and Culture 4
    Continuous Improvement 7
    Cost-Cutting and Value 8
    Lean in Strategy Deployment and Goal Setting 9
    Respect for People 12
Lean Methodology 16
    Continuous Improvement – The PDSA Cycle 18
    A3 Thinking 23
    Value and Non-Value Added Work 33
    Waste 36
    Standardized Work 43
    Leader Standardized Work 46
    Visual Controls 50
    Huddles 53
    The Gemba Walk: How to Lead with Respect 54
    Unevenness and Process Leveling 58
Lean Tools 60
    5S 62
    Five Whys 65
    Fishbone Diagram (Ishikawa Diagram) 69
    Run Chart 70
    Check Sheet 71
    Pareto Chart 72
    Histogram 73
    Scatter Plots 74
    Process Maps 75
    Value Stream Map 76
    Cross-Functional Process Map 80
    Physical Process Map 82
    Communication Maps 83
    Relationship Maps 84
    Generating Ideas from Teams 85

Error-Proofing 89
Getting Started with Lean 92
Getting Ready 94
Lean And QAPI 99
Where to Begin 101
Project Communication (RACI Matrix) 103
Force Field Analysis 104
Gantt Chart 105
Continuous Improvement and Project-Based Improvement 106
Project Components and Structure: A Primer 108
Leadership and Project Sponsorship 109
Managing Change and Encouraging Innovation 111
Practical Strategies for Implementing Change 114
Leading And Lagging Indicators and Process Management 115
Teaching PDSA: The Mr. Potato Head Game 116
PDSA Case Study: Eliminating Alarms From Skilled Nursing Center 117
PDSA Case Study: Reducing Employee Injuries 118
What's Next? 120
Recommended Library for Further Reading 121
Bibliography 122

INTRODUCTION

This is an exciting and challenging time for aging services. Health systems and payers are changing reimbursement models, consumers are demanding better communities and outcomes, and federal regulators continue to increase quality assurance and improvement requirements. In a nutshell, providers must adapt continuously to provide higher quality, more efficient services or risk being left with an empty building or unused services.

Lean is a comprehensive quality improvement strategy, forged from lessons learned across industries, countries, and workplaces. It serves as a cultural anchor, a philosophy of change and a foundation to improve the way you serve residents or clients. But it's more, too: Lean empowers individuals with the tools and ability to listen deeply to residents and create organizations that better serve their needs, now and in the future.

Lean may sound like something that couldn't possibly be of value in aging services. The most common response from providers in this space is, "We're already lean! There's nothing else to cut around here!" It's an understandable reaction in a segment of healthcare that has been deprived of needed resources for decades, while simultaneously being criticized by the media and regulators for not doing enough to care for the persons served. Lean is not, however, about cutting jobs, doing more with less, or trying to squeeze blood from a turnip. Instead, Lean is about doing more of what's important and less of what's not; about doing more that is valuable and less that is wasteful.

Lean is about providing the highest possible value for residents. So, what is value? Essentially, whatever a resident wants and is willing to pay for. In a skilled setting, this means high-quality rehabilitation services, a comfortable environment, and excellent care. In assisted living, this might mean independence and dignity, enabled with support as needed. For home care organizations, value might mean reliable, professional caregivers, proactive support and seamless communication with family members. Sounds like what you already offer, right?

What about mistakes? Errors? Omissions? Have you ever seen any in your community? Mistakes are a type of waste, even if we don't typically think of them that way. Why? Because when a mistake occurs, we have to redo the work. We have to investigate a problem. We have to spend time and money and other resources on something that, in an ideal world, shouldn't have happened in the first place. Ever solve the same problem twice? More waste. Can you look at every person's work at every moment of the day and say with confidence that a resident, with cash in their hand, would be willing to pay for whatever it is the employee is doing? Extra walking, extra charting, extra waiting—there is truly a lot of waste to find. How much? 25%-55% of staff time in skilled nursing is estimated to be spent on wasteful activities. (Petrovich, 2015)

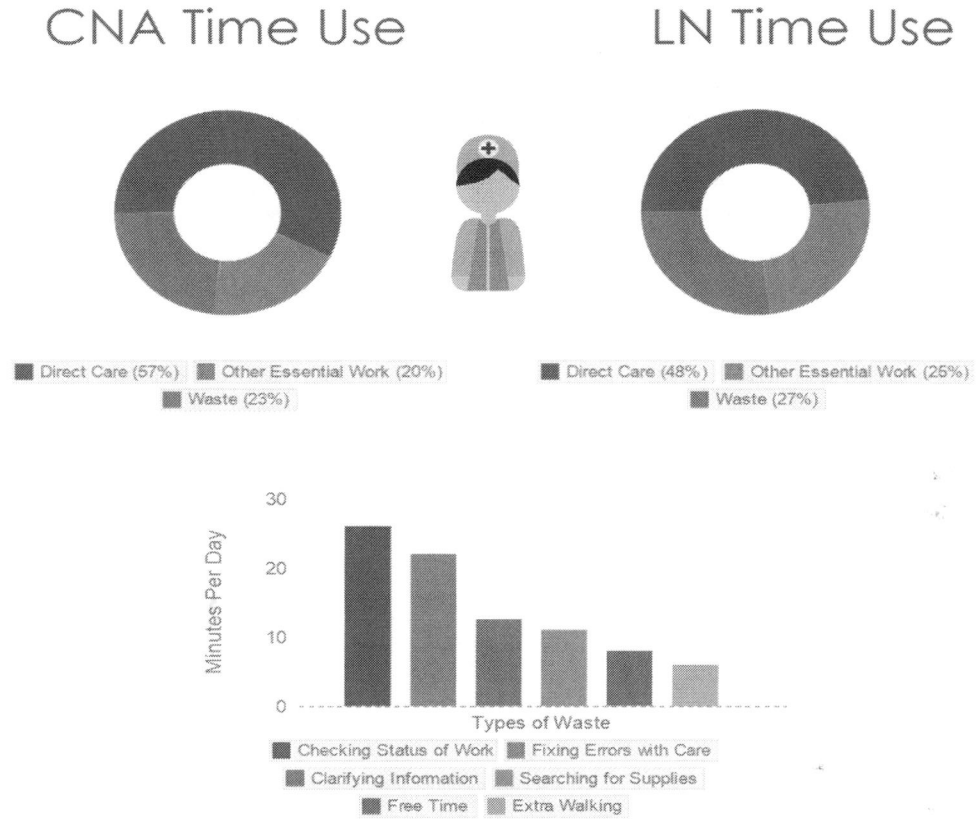

Waste can be difficult to see in healthcare, and especially in aging services, because payment is oftentimes not linked to either quality or value. In addition, an extensive and burdensome regulatory framework encourages waste as a measure of protection against uninhibited surveyors, litigious families, and the impact of an ageist society.

Times are changing, however. Fee-for-service healthcare will soon be an echo of the past, and organizations will instead be judged on (and reimbursed by) how much value they produce. Per diem payments, the RUG payment scheme, and other artifacts of fee-for-service will be replaced by per-episode and capitated payments. Quality is also becoming a component of the payment model, along with outcomes in skilled nursing care. It will no longer be enough to fill beds and deliver therapy—providers will need to demonstrate outstanding quality, high satisfaction, and a relentless approach to increasing value. Under these new conditions, organizations will be unable to cut their way to solutions. Instead, the successful will invest: invest in training, in empowerment, and in continual improvement practices as a way to increase the value of services provided.

Lean is a systemic approach to improvement, and focuses on identifying and eliminating waste (of resources, time, effort, and even human potential) through continuous improvement (in Lean, we say *"kaizen,"* or change for the better) by investing in and empowering everyone in an organization through an engrained philosophy of respect for people. Lean is rooted in the Toyota Production System, and has been successfully deployed in a variety of sectors, including healthcare where efforts have shown significant improvements in quality, safety, efficiency, and employee engagement.

Lean is quickly becoming well established in the healthcare field, and the results have been spectacular: Reduced central line infections by 76% at Allegheny Hospital in Pennsylvania; $54 million in savings through cost reduction and revenue growth at Denver Health in Colorado; reduced readmission for COPD by 48% at UPMC St Margaret in Pennsylvania; reduced patient wait time for orthopedic surgery from 14 weeks to 31 hours at Thedacare in Wisconsin. (Graban, Lean Hospitals, 2012, pp. 5-6) Unfortunately, very little work has addressed the specific challenges and issues in the aging services arena. While this is hardly unexpected—this crucial sector is frequently overlooked in the healthcare continuum—it is doubly unfortunate: First, because resources are already so scarce, and this sector needs to use what it has even more effectively. And second, because Lean focuses resources exactly on the areas of most concern: on value creation, continuous quality improvement (in line with QAPI requirements for nursing homes), and creating a culture of respect for people that can accelerate other culture change and resident-centered improvement initiatives. Lean is truly an embodiment of the work that many of us have been pushing forward for decades.

Lean is sometimes made out to be difficult or hard to master. It isn't. It does take time, true, and there is always more to learn (just as there is always improvements to be made). But if you start simply, build on early gains, and commit to the core tenants and underlying philosophy, you will quickly understand why Lean is a transformational approach to doing work.

There are many fabulous books on Lean and Lean for Healthcare, and I list the titles of several at the end of this one. One challenge I've found with many, though, is they aren't specific enough to aging services—especially for those new to the journey. In this book, I have tried to simplify Lean concepts and apply examples typically found in nursing homes, assisted living communities and other aging services organizations. It's also a combination information guide and workbook, with several tools and guides provided throughout. As you become more familiar with Lean, I highly recommend looking into the wealth of knowledge around Lean Healthcare.

The "culture change" movement, variously named "person-centered care," "resident-centered care," and "person-directed care" is a hot topic for many providers, regulators and consumers. So how does Lean fit in, specifically? As mentioned above, Lean can help accelerate the engagement and respect changes needed to implement culture change ideals. Empowering employees and treating them with respect is something that has eluded many providers for quite some time, despite research that shows such an approach leads to improved resident outcomes. (Anderson, Issel, & McDaniel, 2003) To be successful in the future, we need to rethink many of our long-standing beliefs and traditions. Providers will need to trust employees to do good work by providing appropriate training, adequate support, and ongoing mentorship.

Lean also focuses thinking on the customer's point of view. In fact, the customer is the only one who can define value in a Lean view, and in many cases in aging services, the resident or person served is the ultimate customer. By approaching our services from this perspective, and removing all the other things that aren't wanted or needed, we are able to provide more value with lower cost. And by focusing on underlying respect for people, Lean organizations have higher satisfaction and loyalty scores than other organizations.

A NOTE ON LANGUAGE

Within the Aging Services spectrum, there is currently some debate about words, labels, and their effect on power relations, especially within organizations providing residential and institutional care. In this book, I use the word "community" to refer to an organization, building, facility or nursing home. Likewise, I use the word "neighborhood" to refer to an individual section, unit, or hall within those communities. I use the term "resident" often, though this term can refer to not only a resident of a long-term care community, but also a person served by any organization, such as a senior housing building, a home care agency. I use the term "direct care staff" to denote caregivers, care partners, nursing aides, nurses, and other staff who provide direct services or care to residents.

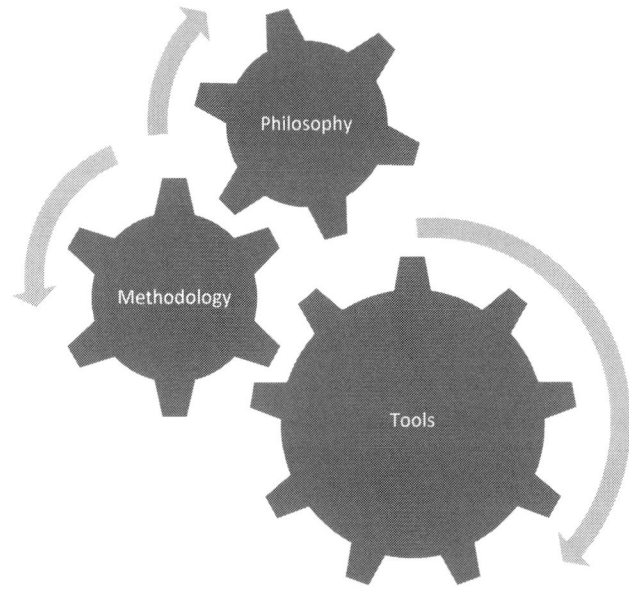

WHAT'S NEXT

The first three sections of the book are devoted to the philosophy, methodology, and common tools of Lean. While tools are the most talked aspect—some may already be familiar to you—they also lead to the least amount of change (just as a large gear does the least amount of work). To drive change faster and more sustainably, be sure to not lose sight of Lean methodology and philosophy when adopting improvement tools.

LEAN PHILOSOPHY

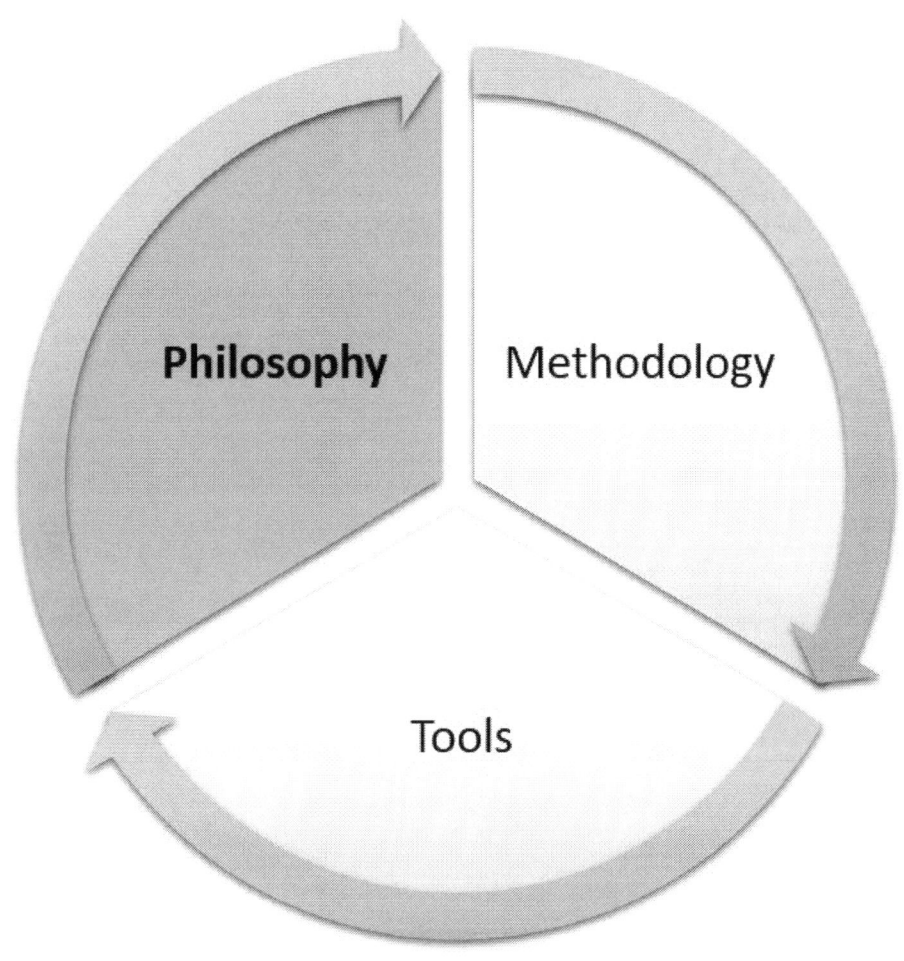

LEAN PHILOSOPHY AND CULTURE

Good care requires good leadership, and good leadership should flow from a thoughtful philosophy about how to serve residents, treat employees, and conduct business.

Lean has simple roots, as you might expect. Sakichi Toyoda, a Japanese serial entrepreneur, owned a large loom factory, specializing in building automatic looms. Automatic looms were a great advance in efficiency, but Toyoda was frustrated by a nagging problem: the machines would continue to work when a thread broke, as if nothing was wrong, causing much of the efficiency to be lost as workers had to unravel the cloth and restart the machine. Diving deep into this irony, he eventually invented a loom that would automatically stop so that an operator would be alerted to a quality problem immediately. This idea of built-in quality (*jidoka*) became central to his budding enterprises. (Rosenthal, 2002)

Let's stop for a second, and think about this. Why is it such a problem for a machine to continue to work after an error? Because you not only have to fix the error, but also redo the work done since. What happens when a CNA makes a basic error in providing care? Perhaps nothing— at least right away. But down the road, the error can lead to an adverse event, a complaint, or a problem to be investigated, documented, and resolved. We rarely think of care mistakes in terms of these costs, and instead have built elaborate systems of oversight and rework to mask the problems—ultimately hiding these costs into the way business is done. It's this compounding and masking of costs that guides Lean's persistent attention to do things right the first time. In manufacturing, rework costs money. In healthcare, it costs money and sometimes much more.

After World War II, Japan's manufacturing base was in shambles, and the automobile industry faced heavy competition from the much more developed operations in Detroit. To make matters worse, Japan faced severe shortages of raw resources. (Womack, 1990, p. 49) Despite these circumstances, Toyota grew to become the largest auto manufacturer in the world. And while American auto manufacturers went through successive bubbles of boom and bust, expanding and laying off workers in cycles, Toyota has steadily grown its business.

Toyota responded to these challenges by creating the Toyota Production System (TPS), developed by executives Taiichi Ohno, Shigeo Shingo, and Kiichiro Toyoda, along with W. Edwards Deming, a quality expert from the United States. (Ohno, 1988, p. 6) Whereas Detroit focused almost entirely on mass production, Toyota's system was built out of the principle of producing high quality products in the most efficient manner possible. Toyota invested in their people, instilled problem solving duties in every position, and focused on making small but constant incremental improvements in processes (*kaizen*). Over time, TPS spread across the world, and across industries, as the principles were adapted to improve operations in software development, service delivery, and healthcare.

So how did Toyota create such a dynamic, successful company?

By combining organizational philosophy, engaged leadership and proven tools in an environment that cultivates success. (Liker, 2004, pp. 37-41)

Lean philosophy can be broken into two foundational ideas:

CONTINUOUS IMPROVEMENT

- Lean is about creating a culture of continuous improvement (*kaizen*) where everyone in the organization looks for opportunities to reduce waste and increase value.
- Value-added processes must be what a customer (resident/ employee/ stakeholder) wants, is willing to pay for, and done right the first time. Non-valued added but necessary processes should be minimized.
- Waste is constantly identified and eliminated. The eight wastes, DOWNTIME, are: Defects, Overproduction, Waiting, Non-utilized talent, Transportation, Inventory, Motion, and Excess processing.

RESPECT FOR PEOPLE

- Managers problem solve by going to the place of work (In Lean, we say *"the gemba"*) and engaging line staff (who best know the work) in creating solutions.
- Organizations provide education, development opportunities, training and necessary resources to effectively empower workers and create exceptional employees.
- Care is taken to not over-burden and over-work staff, as this leads to resentment, low morale, poor quality and employee injuries.

Lean focuses on creating value. As a philosophy, Lean promotes leadership connected to the place of work, builds teams of problem solvers, shares information freely and openly, and creates processes and systems with quality hardwired.

Lean is principle and process-focused. Toyota believes that ordinary people, working with extraordinary processes, can do great work. Conversely, extraordinary people working with ordinary processes will produce only average results. Deming, reflecting on his extensive career in quality management, noted that approximately 94% of problems belong to the system (and thus the responsibility of management) and only 6% to human factors. (Deming, 2000, p. 315) Contrast this view to what we oftentimes find in aging services, where individuals are usually held responsible for problems and errors.

In many long-term care organizations, management focuses on accountability and oversight of people rather than processes. It's no wonder we spend so much time trying to fix problems—we're focusing on the wrong things! In the traditional view, supervision of staff is paramount, and considerable time is spent ensuring policies and procedures are followed. Administrators spend a lot of time in their offices, reviewing incident reports, census reports, quality reports, et cetera. Meanwhile, staff are engaged in the work of caring for residents, frequently without enough supplies, tools or training to complete their job duties. Inevitably, this arrangement leads to challenges with quality and compliance, and precious time is wasted on fixing recurrent problems and constantly fighting fires.

Lean organizations approach quality through proactive system building. Managers cannot stay in their offices to be successful. Instead, they must spend considerable time in work areas, coaching, challenging and learning from line staff.

	Traditional LTC Leadership	**Lean Leadership**
Focus	Compliance with standards; Month-to month financials; managing individual components to promote quality	Value (Best quality with lowest cost); long-term view; looking at system-wide processes and performance
Approach	Supervision, Positional Authority	Coaching, Mentoring, Deep support
Training of staff	Minimum necessary; most training is done in classrooms	Substantial; most training is done on the floor during work
Response to problems	Supervisor investigates; policy and procedure change; in-services; disciplinary action	Supervisor assists and challenges staff; root cause analysis; counter-measures; error-proofing
Staff Engagement	Superficial, irregular	High, expected of all employees
Labor-Management Relations	Adversarial, based on independent goals and finite resources.	Collaborative, based on mutual respect and trust. Focused on success of all parties.
Long-term Growth	Challenging; most time is spent fighting fires and recurrent problems	Sustainable; work is constantly improved, building capacity for future challenges

CONTINUOUS IMPROVEMENT

In Lean, the word *kaizen* means "change for the better" and describes a systemic and continuous approach to improving work. Many organizations, of course, have ongoing efforts to improve their offerings and service, with varying levels of success. For Lean organizations, continuous improvement is a structured, resourced, and managed process that occurs throughout an organization. It is rooted in ongoing problem solving and solution testing and built on the understanding that practices must continually be improved to keep up with changing knowledge, technology and resident needs.

To build a culture of continuous improvement, it is first important to remove the notion that improvement work is only the job of certain positions or committees; everyone must participate and be supported for an organization to succeed. Each position in an organization needs to be allotted with some time for reflection and improvement work on a regular basis. Some organizations structure this time around slower periods of the day or at shift change.

Building the culture of improvement should start even before employees are hired. Give prospective team members information about your organization's continuous improvement program, and ask them about their comfort and willingness to participate in helping the organization better serve residents. Once hired, it is imperative that orientation includes additional information on improvement knowledge and expectations. Make sure that new employees also know where to go for help and support.

Improvement efforts and areas of opportunity also need to be clearly communicated so that progress can be tracked and supported. Using tools like the A3 problem solving document and visual management like a "How Are We Doing Board" help to accomplish this.

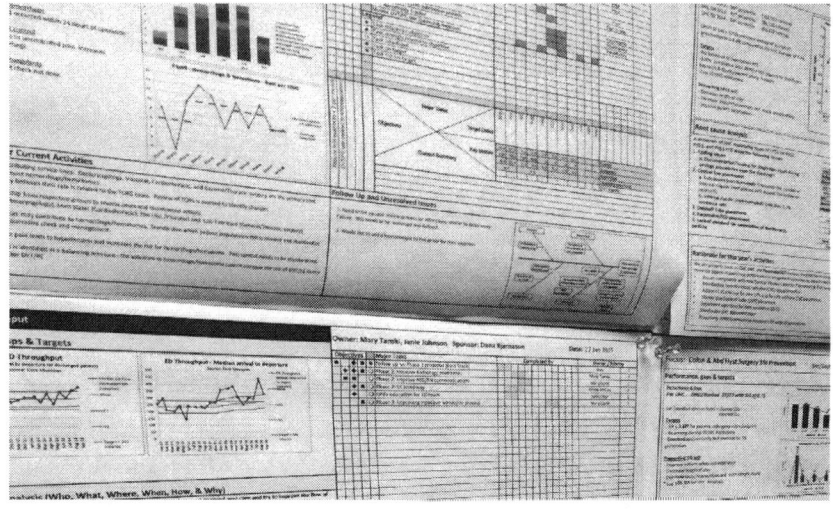

Example of a How Are We Doing Board

COST-CUTTING AND VALUE

There is no doubt that tough times are ahead in aging services. For years, organizations have tried to reduce expenses, expand services lines and find pennies hidden in the pavement. In many communities, it's almost hard to imagine things could be "leaned" any more. Lean, however, provides a very different approach to the problem of limited resources than traditional cost-cutting does. Rather than focus on costs as the main problem, Lean focuses on waste—the part of cost that doesn't add value to what you offer. Waste appears in many forms—we'll dive deeper into that later—but the key to long-term growth and sustainability is relentlessly pursuing its elimination.

Say you need a new Hoyer lift. Should you buy the one that's $2,500 or the one that's $4,000? That's not enough information, you might say. You might want to know, does the $4,000 last longer? Does it have a higher weight capacity? Does it include a maintenance contract? All of these factors adjust the "value" of the lift. If you focus solely on cost, the $2,500 lift is better than the $4,000. But if it breaks quicker or doesn't do the job you need it to do, it may not be a better value.

The same is true for other "costs"—like employees. Organizations sometimes spend enormous efforts to manage incremental overtime (the 15 minutes at the end of a shift) or schedule shift employees for 7.5 hours to eliminate overlap, thinking that these approaches help to save money. While they may reduce costs, these efforts also impact quality, engagement and satisfaction and can lead to lower overall value. Without shift overlap, for example, communication between shifts is difficult (if not impossible at times), leading to care gaps and potential resident harm. Managing incremental overtime across the board causes employees to take shortcuts or push off work onto the next shift, leading to lower morale, shift-to-shift conflicts, and care issues.

During tough times, an organization may try to reduce costs by some measure (say, a 5% reduction) across all departments, usually to avoid bickering between department heads or divisions. Unfortunately, broad cuts affect value activities almost as much as they affect waste activities. In typical fashion, given time, costs inevitably rise—usually because of shortcuts, deferred maintenance, or resident complaints. In some cases, like new hire orientation and training, cost-cutting on the front-end leads to significant increased costs over time. Despite significant research on the costs and causes of turnover, it remains stubbornly high in aging services, again because of the attention to cost over value. (Kayyali, 2014 Sep) (Mukamel, Spector, Limcangco, & et al., 2009)

To be successful over time, we must shift our focus to value rather than costs. Instead of viewing investments in employee training, wages, and supplies as costs, look at them in terms of impact on resident care, satisfaction, and over efficiency of operations.

LEAN IN STRATEGY DEPLOYMENT AND GOAL SETTING

Goal setting can be very difficult in aging services because of the constant attention to urgent needs and crises. Even when time is found to spend on strategic planning, the results oftentimes end up sitting in a binder on a shelf or locked away in a storage closet. Line staff, well-versed in the empty talk of management, learn to gloss over any suggestion of a new idea or program, content to wait and see if this one will miraculously stick.

Lean practices a form of goal setting that relies on strong involvement of everyone in the organization. While senior management determines the overall vision and direction for the organization, middle management works on specific strategy and projects to implement the vison through a shared process of goal-setting. Line staff, then, organize the work and implement plans based on jointly established measures. Finally, senior management completes the loop by reviewing the execution of staff and making adjustments or providing support as necessary. (Akao, 2004, p. XXV)

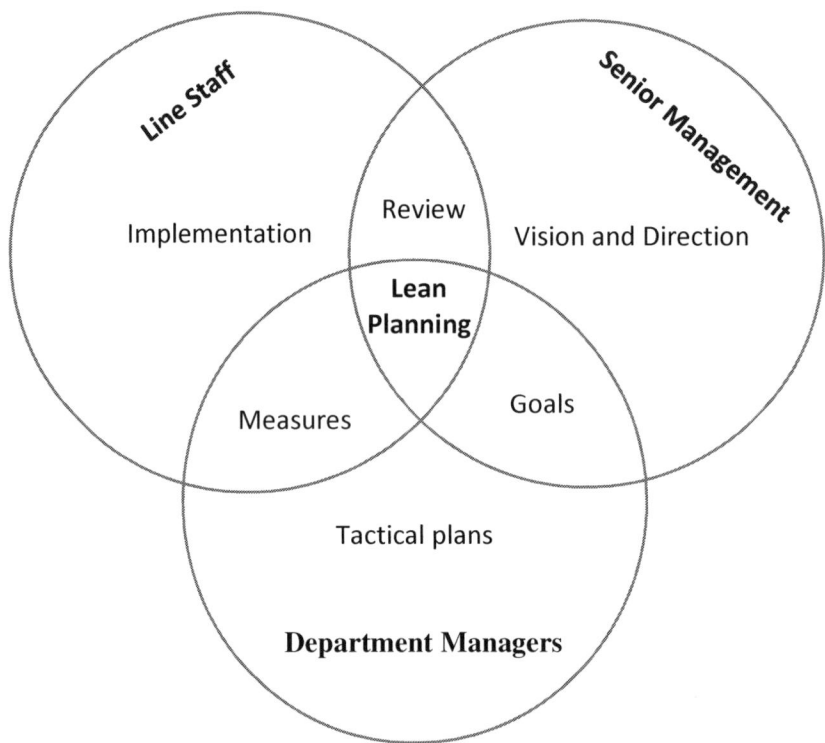

When plans are being developed, they should travel back and forth along lines of authority, with senior leaders seeking input from department managers and line staff and making revisions based on this feedback. This process, sometimes called "catchball" because of its relation to passing a ball back and forth, promotes bi-directional dialogue and ownership.

This helps to ensure goals are in line with actual challenges on the ground, as well as builds information and support from line staff regarding organizational priorities. Many a management goal has been stalled or thwarted because of a lack of support and action from employees. By making goal setting and actualization a collaborative, dynamic process, you not only come up with better goals—you increase the likelihood of meeting them.

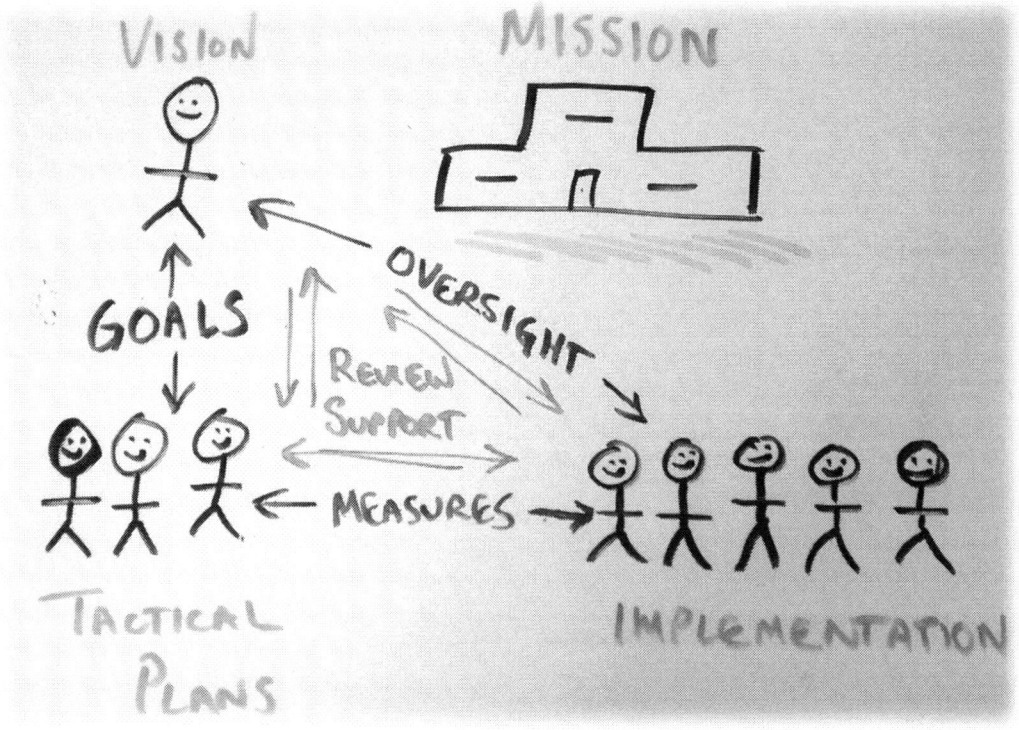

1. Senior leadership develops the overall vision ("What are we doing?"), based on the mission of the organization.
2. Senior leadership and mid-level managers jointly develop goals ("Where are we going?"), based on the vision.
3. Mid-level managers develop tactical plans ("How will we get there?"), based on goals.
4. Mid-level managers and line staff develop measures ("How will we know when we get there?"), based on the tactical plans.
5. Line staff develop and execute implementation plans ("What work do we need to accomplish to get there?"), based on measures.
6. Senior leadership reviews the execution of implementation plans for alignment with the vision, mission, and appropriate time tables.

Note: Ongoing review and support occurs continuously throughout the organization.

X Diagram (Hoshin Kanri / Policy Deployment)

Annual Objectives (Top):
- Foundation Fund to $500K by FYE
- Launch Home Care Division to all On-Campus Residents
- Operating Cash Flow Ratio to 100% by FYE

Key Initiatives (3-5 Years) (Left):
- Foundation Fund to $1MM by 2015
- CF Positive Home Care Division by 2015
- Operating Cash Flow Ratio to 102% by 2014

Tactical Strategies (Right):
- Increase Rental Revenue
- Reduce Apartment Turnover Time
- Develop Home Care Business
- Develop Internal Business Processes for Home Care Division
- Create Foundation Entity

Measurable Targets to Achieve (Bottom):
- Increase Rental Income to $65K monthly
- Reduce apartment turnover from 22 days to 15 days
- Increase intent list applicants by 10%
- Complete Home Care Certification Process
- Pilot Home Care Division to Towers
- Expand Home Care Pilot to Villas
- Hire Foundation Director
- Allocate funds to Foundation during budgeting process

Key Personnel Accountable:
- CEO
- CFO
- VP Clinical Services
- VP Resident Relations

The X diagram (part of *Hoshin Kanri*, or Policy Deployment), is a useful tool that links initiatives to actionable targets. Begin on the left side with key initiatives, and work clockwise around the document to develop annual objectives, tactical strategies, measureable targets and personnel accountable. Use the boxes in the corners to show linkages. This document is a visual way to help an organization progress towards strategic goals.

RESPECT FOR PEOPLE

Most organizations would say they respect their employees. And in some senses, this is true. Following laws and regulations, offering opportunities for growth and advancement, providing a workplace free from harassment, and paying competitive wages and benefits are the most common ways that organizations show their respect.

In Lean, respect means much, much more. Respect for people means that employees are not over-burdened by work. It means that employees are expected to be engaged problem solvers and active participants so that their natural skills and talents as humans are not wasted. Respect means that employees are listened to—and even encouraged to bring up potential problems they notice. It means that employee safety is a top management concern. From this view, there is obviously a lot more that Aging Services organizations can do.

Protecting employees from being over-burdened by work, what the Japanese call *muri*, or unreasonableness, is worth particular attention, since overwork leads to a host of problems, including mistakes, shortcuts, burnout and employee turnover. A useful exercise to consider is writing out all of the work expected of a particular position, along with the time it takes to complete the work. For a CNA, for example, write out all the tasks they are expected to complete with the time it takes to do the task properly. When added together, it's common to find the list of tasks takes much more time than the standard shift would allow, and provides a good starting place for examining areas of waste and opportunities for improvement.

Perhaps you have heard the phrase, "The beatings will continue until morale improves." This, unfortunately, is a philosophy far too common in long-term care organizations. When mistakes occur, line staff are frequently blamed and counseled to "do better" or "try harder" or "be more careful." Focused training is provided after an error occurs, and employees who "don't get it" are shown the door. Some organizations are in near-constant crisis, and everyone is expected to keep their head down and not mention any additional problems they may notice. There is barely enough time to fix the challenges that are known, so there is little reason to look for more.

For quality to improve, organizations must eliminate this punitive atmosphere and focus on system assessment and improving design instead. Remember Demings' observation that 94% of errors are system-induced, not the fault of people? If we look carefully, we see that most errors in healthcare are caused by system failures—whether lack of training, broken equipment, not enough time, management incompetence—and they will only be sustainably fixed when organizations stop focusing on individuals as the source of problems and look at the whole system instead.

This is different than simply not holding staff accountable for their actions, however. "Just Culture," a growing movement in healthcare that aligns well with Lean's respect for people, provides a good framework for appropriately placing accountability. Just Culture separates out errors into system issues, negligent behavior and willful conduct, and recommends appropriate action based on the cause. Why is this important? Because while system design will guide staff behavior, individuals still make choices. Some choices, such as the willful disregard of workable safety procedures, are very different from others, such as having to choose between competing safety procedures because of a lack of resources.

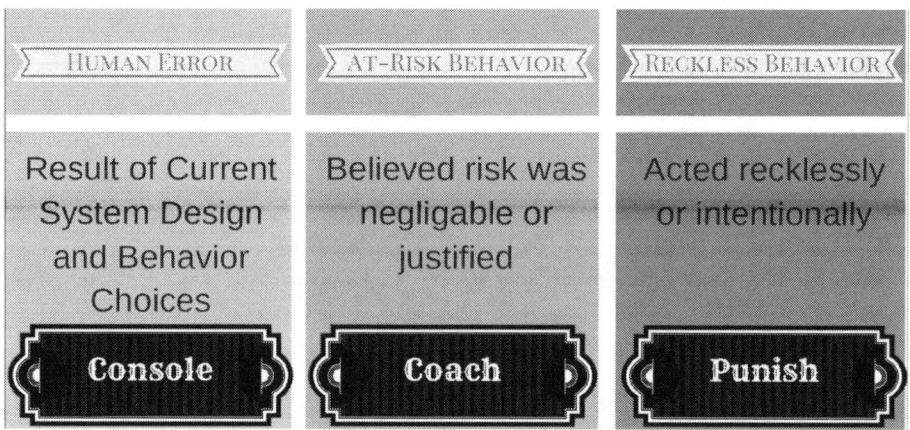

To determine the cause, consider whether the behavior was intended, whether safety procedures were knowingly violated, whether practices were actually workable (i.e., the employee had access to the right equipment, supplies, and time necessary), whether another employee, in the same situation, would have had the same result, and whether there is a history of similar behavior.

Decision Tree for Accountability

Decision flow

- **Were the actions as intended?**
  - No → Did the individual knowingly violate policies/protocols or safe procedures?
  - Yes → **Were the consequences as intended?**
    - Yes → Sabotage, malevolent damage
    - No → Did the individual knowingly violate policies/protocols or safe procedures?

- **Did the individual knowingly violate policies/protocols or safe procedures?**
  - Yes → Were standard practices and procedures available, workable, correct and in routine use?
    - No → Would another individual, with similar experience and training, behave similarly?
    - Yes → Were the expectations known, reasonable, and understood?
      - No → Would another individual, with similar experience and training, behave similarly?
      - Yes → Is there evidence that the individual took an unacceptable risk?
  - No → Would another individual, with similar experience and training, behave similarly?

- **Would another individual, with similar experience and training, behave similarly?**
  - Yes → Does the individual have a history of unsafe acts?
  - No → Were there deficiencies in tools, training, experience or supervision?
    - Yes → Does the individual have a history of unsafe acts?
    - No → Is there evidence that the individual took an unacceptable risk?

- **Is there evidence that the individual took an unacceptable risk?**
  - Yes → Were there significant mitigating circumstances?
    - Yes → Does the individual have a history of unsafe acts?
    - No → Possible reckless violation
  - No → Possible negligent behavior

- **Does the individual have a history of unsafe acts?**
  - Yes → System induced error, with training indicated
  - No → System induced/blameless error

Outcomes (left to right)

- Sabotage, malevolent damage
- Possible reckless violation
- Possible negligent behavior
- System induced error, with training indicated
- System induced/blameless error

Individual Accountability ———————————————— **Organization Accountability**

Starting at the beginning, determine if the actions were intended. If yes, determine if the consequences were intended. Generally, the answer to at least one of these questions is no. Staff generally don't intentionally cause harm or create a negative outcome. In the case where both answers are yes, the employee committed an intentional error; take immediate action proportionate to the action and outcome.

Third, determine if policies or safety procedures were knowingly violated. If yes, were the procedures reasonable, available, and doable? It's crucial to really examine those procedures to make sure they are workable: do staff have enough time and resources to follow them? You may find that expectations aren't reasonable, and must be adjusted for staff to reliably do good work. If procedures were reasonable, the employee may have committed a reckless error. Provide counseling or corrective action, based on the employee's performance history.

If policies weren't reasonable, or not regularly followed by staff, determine if someone else, with similar training and experience, placed in a similar situation, would produce the same result. This is called the "substitution test." If the answer is no, review the training and experience of the employee and determine if deficiencies were present. If deficiencies are present, offer the necessary training to remedy the situation and provide coaching to ensure future compliance. If the employee had the appropriate training and experience, the error was a potentially negligent action, and you should provide counseling or corrective action, based on the employee's performance history.

Finally, review if the employee has a history of unsafe acts. If they have, the error itself may be blameless (it could have happened to anyone), but additional training or coaching may be warranted based on the employee's history. If not, the error is blameless and the employee should be consoled regarding the error: it could have happened to any staff member, and it was caused by a system failure, not an individual one. The error should be reviewed to determine how error-proofing can be applied to prevent future occurrences.

Following this model, you will see that most errors and mistakes that occur are either system-induced or blameless errors. It's crucial to develop an atmosphere that respects employees for the work they do, and work actively to create systems and practices that support those employees in making good choices.

LEAN METHODOLOGY

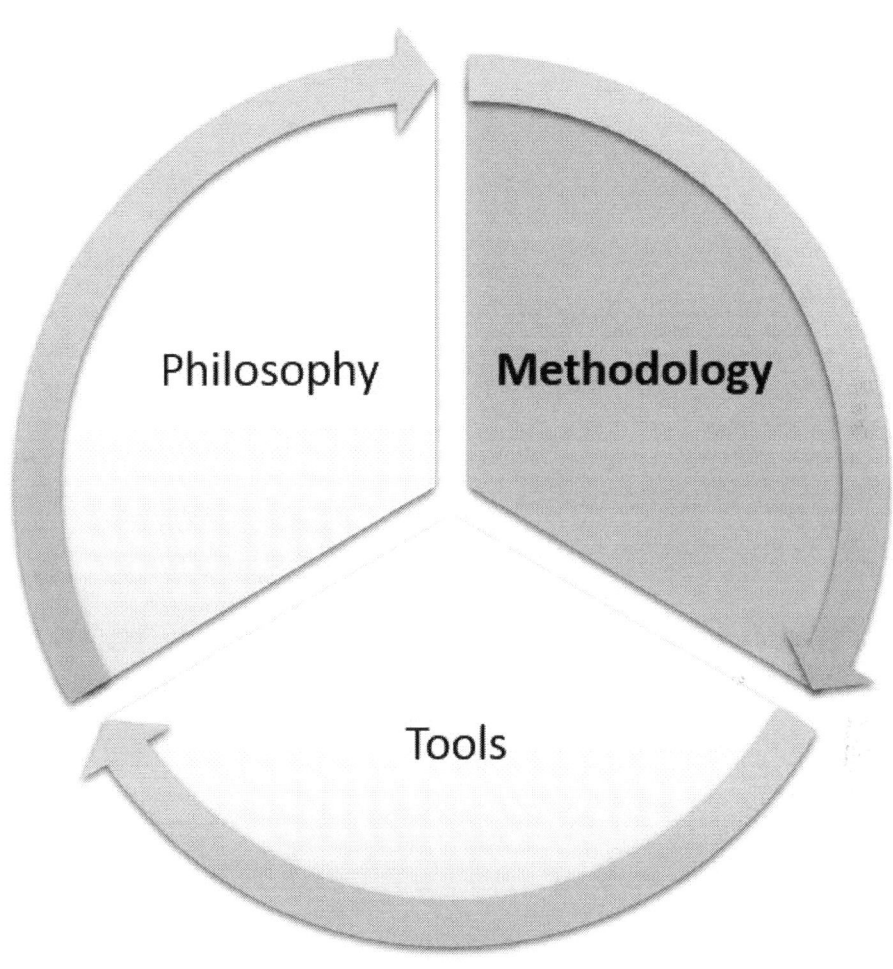

CONTINUOUS IMPROVEMENT – THE PDSA CYCLE

Dr. Edwards Deming is credited with developing the Plan-Do-Study-Act (PDSA) cycle of continuous quality improvement based on his learning from Walter Shewhart at Bell Labs. The cycle is also known as Plan-Do-Check-Act (PDCA), the Shewhart cycle, or the Deming Wheel, and is based on the scientific method. The Institute for Healthcare Improvement (IHI), a leading healthcare improvement and advocacy organization, developed a similar model called the Model for Improvement, which adds the questions, "What are we trying to accomplish?," "How will we know that a change is an improvement?," and "What changes can we make that will result in improvement?" (Improvement, 2014) Six Sigma is another improvement methodology becoming common in healthcare organizations. As you can see, all of the problem solving strategies follow the same basic principles.

Problem Solving Methodologies

Validate the Problem	Access/ Focus the Problem	Learn/ Verify Root Causes	Change/ Evaluate Process	Verify Improvement	Sustain Gains

Scientific Method

Ask a Question	Background Research	Form Hypothesis	Conduct Experiment	Analyze Results	Share Findings

PDSA

Plan	Do	Study	Act

IHI Model for Improvement

Plan: Aim, Measures, Ideas	Do	Study	Act

Six Sigma

Define	Measure	Analyze	Improve	Control

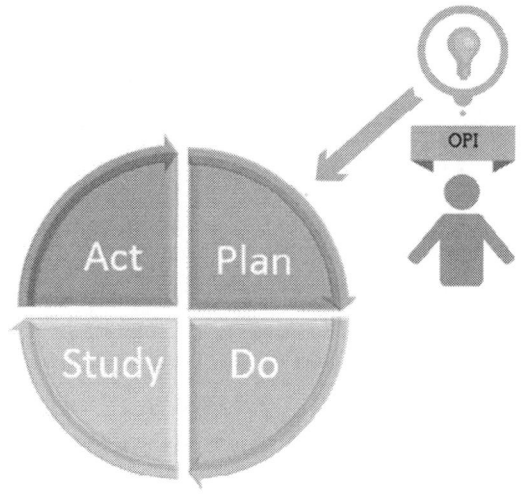

The PDSA cycle begins with an opportunity for process improvement (OPI). This is a problem, an error, or an area you've identified as needing improvement.

Where do you get ideas? From residents! From families! From employees! Regular satisfaction and engagement surveys are a great start. Informal coffee hours, "Lunch with the Administrator" programs, and regular time spent on the floor with staff are also crucial avenues for feedback. In care environments with regular care or service planning meetings, be sure to engage participants in understanding not only care needs, but also their overall experience and any frustrations they experience.

OPI boards are a great way to engage staff, too. Staff can post ideas and share projects in process. The key to success, however, is a clear chain to beginning experiments. Anyone can have an idea, but if it is never tested or implemented, people quickly learn to stop making suggestions. Indeed, this is the biggest challenge with "suggestion boxes" and the like: an idea goes in, and then nothing happens. It's important to create a short, responsive chain to trying out suggestions quickly.

Mark Graban, who works with the improvement software *KaiNexus*, describes how a kaizen system is different:

> "[W]e encourage people to start small. Instead of a funnel that winnows things down to the best idea, Kaizen casts a wide net. We can have dozens or hundreds of ideas being implemented in parallel. We don't need to run each idea all the way up the flagpole for approval at the very senior levels of management.
>
> In an 'idea management' approach, people will get discouraged when their good ideas aren't accepted for implementation. With Kaizen, people are allowed to make local decisions as ideas 'bubble up.' " (Graban, Will Suggestion Boxes be a Trend in 2012? What Method(s) do we Need for Employee Engagement?, 2011)

At Toyota, employees submit an average of 4 suggestions per month, and an astounding 96% of these ideas were implemented. Between 1948 and 1988, Toyota estimated its employees generated 20 million ideas for improvement! Even more importantly, Toyota budgets 50% of the team leader's time to encouraging and testing employee ideas. (Protzman, Mayzell, & Kerpchar, 2011, p. 52)

PLAN

Once you have an idea, you can begin the improvement cycle. In the planning phase, clearly identify the problem, establish a baseline, develop an understanding of what the future state should look like (once the problem has been removed), and conduct a root cause analysis to determine the likely cause or causes of the problem.

It is not uncommon for a problem to begin somewhat vague. A staff member might report that there are never enough washcloths available, or a resident might complain that her coffee is cold. Further investigation might reveal that the true problem is not only washcloths, but other laundry products as well, or only regular coffee and not decaf. By clarifying the problem early on in the process, further work will be both more accurate and more likely to result in sustained improvement.

Collecting baseline data is crucial for two reasons: first, you need to validate the problem and understand its extent. Some problems seem worse than they actually are, while other problems are more prevalent than they seem; collecting baseline data helps ensure improvement effects are focused on the most important and impactful issues. Second, baseline data allows you to compare the situation before and after trying an intervention to know whether changes had any effect on the problem. Too often, organizations will apply a solution without regard to whether it actually makes a difference. Baseline data for some problems might be readily available, such as incident numbers or rehospitalizations. Other problems might require a collection period where staff observe or record how often a problem occurs.

After collecting baseline data, begin to examine the causes of the problem, drilling down to understand the true root causes. Common tools (explained later in more detail) include the five whys, fishbone diagrams, run charts, trend reports and process maps.

Once the likely root cause or causes have been identified, identify solutions or countermeasures that can be tested. (Lean prefers the term "countermeasure" over "solution" because most systems and processes are so complex and change often enough that there is rarely a permanent solution; instead, we implement countermeasures to the likely causes of a problem to lower the risk that a problem will occur. In addition, thinking about countermeasures as opposed to solutions encourages a mindset of continuous improvements to a process rather than a goal to reach and then forget about.)

Use the following hypothesis statement to evaluate countermeasures: If we *(countermeasure)*, then *(root cause)* won't occur/ will occur less often.

DO

In the do phase of the cycle, test out the proposed countermeasures. It's usually best to trial countermeasures in a limited area first, such as one neighborhood or department, so you can make modifications or adjustments before rolling it out to the whole community. Before you begin, be sure you have a plan to collect data on effectiveness of the interventions and a timeline to review that data. Also, include a review of staff or resident reception and collect information on any ways that the implementation could have gone better—this is crucial for making larger rollouts more successful.

STUDY

After implementing countermeasures, analyze the results of the data collected from the pilot tests. Were the countermeasures effective? Is the problem better? Worse? The same? Different changes can require different timelines for checking on their effectiveness, but generally 30, 60 and 90 day marks provide a good place to check on the status of countermeasures.

It's not uncommon to fall into the trap of the "Plan-Do" cycle, where problem solving and action are followed by forgetting about an issue until it pops up again. Many forms and procedures have been created after an initial problem analysis and are quickly implemented, but are never evaluated to see if they are actually effective. The study phase is a crucial link between initial hypothesis testing and sustained results—indeed, this is the key to actual improvements that sustain over time.

Two of the biggest hurdles to following through with an evaluation are a lack of time and a fear of failure. To overcome these hurdles, develop the understanding that implementing a countermeasure is only half of the work cycle. Ensure that pilot programs are evaluated before being expanded and that action plans include a study/ review component in their planned timeline.

In addition to collecting data on the test, it is important to determine if the test occurred as planned. Sometimes, unforeseen variables creep into an experiment and these must be accounted for during an evaluation. Other times, it may be more difficult than planned to collect data and it might be necessary to make an early adjustment to the test.

ACT

If countermeasures were found to be effective, incorporate any improvements or learning from the pilot and roll out the countermeasures to other appropriate areas. It's crucial to solidify gains and ensure they become part of updated work guidelines and training. Significant duplication of efforts occurs when countermeasures aren't continued and the problem re-occurs, or—especially in larger communities—when one neighborhood adopts an improved practice, but others continue to struggle with the root problem.

What happens if the changes didn't produce the desired results? First, don't worry! Thomas Edison is credited with saying, "I did not fail 1000 times. I did not fail once. I merely found 1000 ways that didn't work." Similarly, scientists at the Rocket Chemical Company in 1953 failed thirty nine times to create a water displacement product before reaching the formula we now know as WD-40®. (The WD-40 Company, n.d.)

Finding out what doesn't work is just as important as finding out what does, but it takes confidence and perseverance to continue on. Be sure to support and reassure staff when pilots don't turn out as expected. Building confidence in using the PDSA cycle can take time, but the benefits far outweigh the initial fear of being wrong or making a mistake.

When analyzing a failed test, it is important to separate out a test that showed an intervention was unsuccessful from a test that wasn't conducted successfully. For a test that wasn't conducted successfully, consider the following questions:

- Was the pilot successfully launched?
- Were area staff involved effectively?
- Was there a data collection problem?
- Were unknown variables introduced during the implementation?

After addressing these questions, you may consider rerunning the pilot. On the other hand, if a pilot determines that an intervention wasn't successful, consider these questions:

- Was a root cause incorrect or missing?
- Did the pilot identify unknown barriers to implementing the countermeasure?
- Would the countermeasure be more effective if paired with an additional intervention?

At this point, it is crucial to take the learnings from the test and restart the PDSA cycle.

The key to the PDSA cycle is to work methodically through challenges, experiment with and evaluate changes, and act on the results. The cycle is never truly "done"— you'll always be able to improve or fine-tune a process. Indeed, it is key to remember this is a *cycle*. Many of the problems with improvements that fail to take hold can be traced to improper attention to the PDSA process. (Taylor, McNicolas, Nicolay, & Darzi, 2013)

Organizations need to also ensure that their performance review process and compensation plans promote experimenting and continuous learning and not just quick fixes or short-term results. Focusing solely on outcomes, rather than underlying processes, is a sure way to develop an unstable and unsustainable organization.

A3 THINKING

PDSA is the basis for A3 thinking, a tool that grounds the improvement cycle in an easier to understand and follow process. By working through problems and their causes in a scientific, methodical way, we can develop effective countermeasures and build on prior success.

A3 thinking is an important Lean problem solving practice. The name "A3" comes from the metric size of paper, approximately 11"x17", which is used to develop the A3 report. Toyota developed the A3 format as a systemic problem-solving approach based on PDSA. The scope of a problem being addressed should fit onto the page. This is one way the A3 helps to protect against trying to solve too many problems or too big a problem at once—if it won't fit, try reducing the scope. (Since A3 paper size isn't as common here, you can use two sheets of 8 ½x 11. A sample template is provided at the end of this section.) A3s should also ideally be written in pencil. That way, you can easily erase and make changes as you learn.

An A3 serves as both a problem solving tool and a report of the problem solving activity, typically used to communicate project success to stakeholders and leadership. Why is this crucial? Because we sometimes waste a great deal of time fixing problems only to find out later that some neighborhood, shifts, or staff members didn't know about the updated policy or practice. With a visual guide to the problem and effective countermeasures, we begin the work of building strong and reliable standards into practice.

A3 reports cannot be completed in an office or conference room, nor can they be completed by a supervisor or manager alone. Rather, representatives from the entire team involved must participate, and the work should be based on actual observations of the problem site. For instance, if you are trying to resolve an issue with lift slings, you must gather CNAs, charge nurses and laundry staff together, and physically go to the storage and laundry areas. By problem solving in this hands-on fashion, you will be much more likely to identify true root cause issues and develop workable and sustainable countermeasures.

The A3 can be easily broken down into nine components or sections:

1. **Reason for action**. This contains the problem statement (the gap between where you are and where you want to be, addressing the what, when, who, where and how much), the importance statement (what's the rationale for fixing the problem? why is it important to the organization?), and the project scope (what parts of the process are included in the problem and what parts are excluded). This is particularly important with issues that may take significant time to resolve.

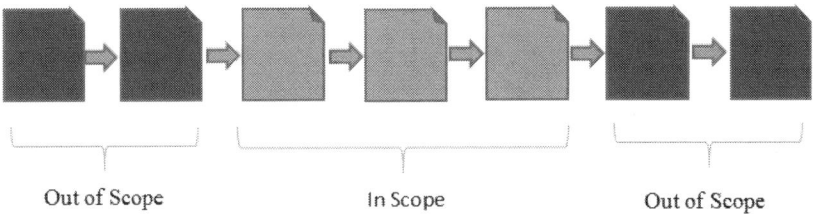

Out of Scope   In Scope   Out of Scope

Determining the right scope of an issue to tackle in an A3 is crucial: too small and the problem may be fragmented or sub-optimized; too big and the root cause(s) will be unclear or too many to address.

2. **Current state**. Write out or draw the current process, including any data you've collected that validates the problem (how long a process takes, how many errors occur). To do this, visit the work area and observe the actual process. Review the work with staff members. It's very important that the current state reflects the work that is actually occurring, not the work you think is occurring.

   Capturing the current state can sometimes be challenging, particularly in communities where trust is strained or absent. When collecting information from line staff, be sure not to be critical of how they are doing the work—if it is different than what you expect, there is probably a reason. Uncovering that reason becomes part of the problem solving process.

   When problem areas in the current state are known, draw storm clouds and label the issues. This becomes a visual cue of the areas to focus thinking.

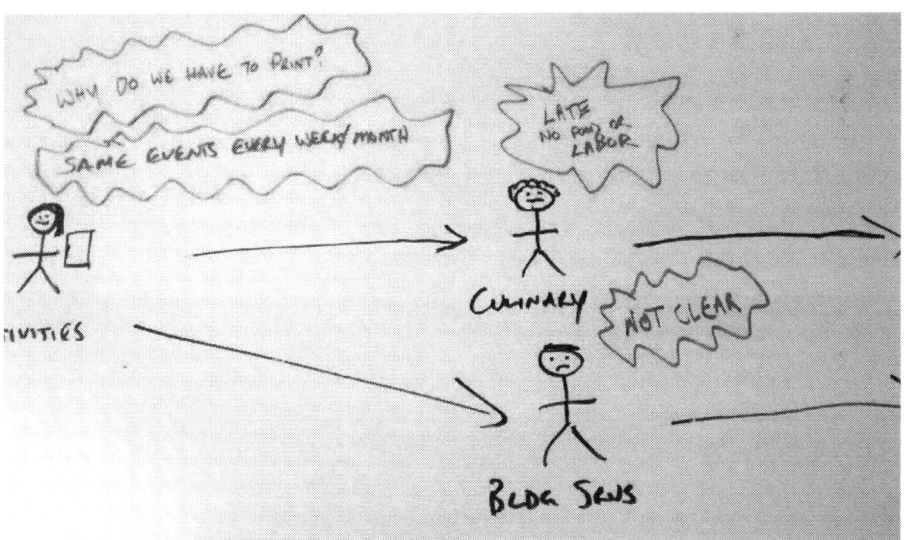

Portion of a current state drawing, with problem areas written in the cloud objects

24

3. **Goal state**. Write out or draw the future process. What does a better functioning system look like? (Include goals relating to the metrics measured in the current state.) Note, this is not simply the absence of the problem, but rather, what would good look like?

4. **Root cause analysis**. Identify reasons for the problem occurring. Use problem solving tools like the five whys or a fishbone diagram to seek out the true root causes. It's important to not get caught up in trying to quickly solve the problem by addressing only superficial causes. If a root cause is "staff member made a mistake" or "staff member didn't follow the plan of care or policy/procedure," you're still

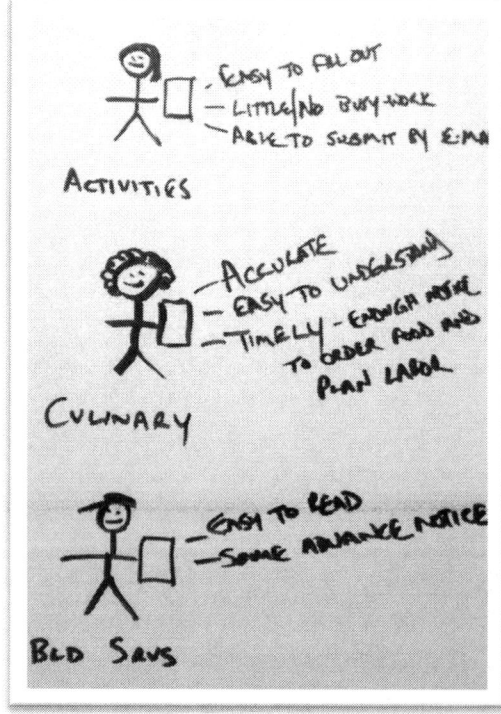

Portion of the goal state drawing

at the surface of the problem; keep digging to find the underlying causes. (See the Lean Tools section for help with this process.)

5. **Solution/ Countermeasure approach**. Brainstorm countermeasures (solutions) to the root causes identified. Make sure solutions are tied to the identified root causes; otherwise, you will waste energy implementing changes that will have little to no impact. Here again, be very cautious if your solution is to re-issue a policy/ procedure or retrain a single staff member; while occasionally this may be a useful intervention, usually problems require deeper or more expansive interventions. (For instance, if an employee is unaware of the correct procedure, are there visual aids that could be added to make the work more transparent? Are your training practices sufficient? Is there underlying team challenges that are stifling communication?)

6. **Testing and pilot projects**. Test out the countermeasures in a particular area or unit and measure the results. Did the changes lead to the results expected? If not, return to the root cause analysis and solution/ countermeasure phases to identify additional or different causes and countermeasures.

7. **Implementation/ completion plans**. When countermeasures have been verified, identify who will implement them across needed areas. Be specific in listing the

action, person responsible and timeline for implementation. This makes actions clear to all involved, and helps to ensure accountability to try the countermeasures.

8. **Confirm gains**. Be sure to monitor and record progress on the issue for 30-90 days afterwards to ensure the countermeasures have been effective. It's important that line staff understand it's okay if countermeasures don't work. Worse than trying something that doesn't work is continuing to do it forever, so it's important to discontinue ineffective interventions and return to the root cause analysis.

9. **Insights/ lessons to share**. Document any important learnings that can be shared across the organization. Remember, one of the important functions of the A3 report is to circulate learning across departments and demonstrate to staff that identifying problems can result in improvements to the workplace. Ideally, create a wall to hang completed A3s as reminders of the hard work and changes made.

Optional: Cost analysis. Some organizations like to include a cost analysis of the interventions and the potential savings when the problem is avoided. This helps to justify equipment purchases and system changes, and can be used to support the value of Lean work. If you decide not to record this on the A3 form, make sure it's tracked somewhere, especially at the beginning of a Lean journey. It can be crucial to show the value of savings early on, and some organizations use a rolling number posted in the staff break room to remind staff how valuable improvement work truly is.

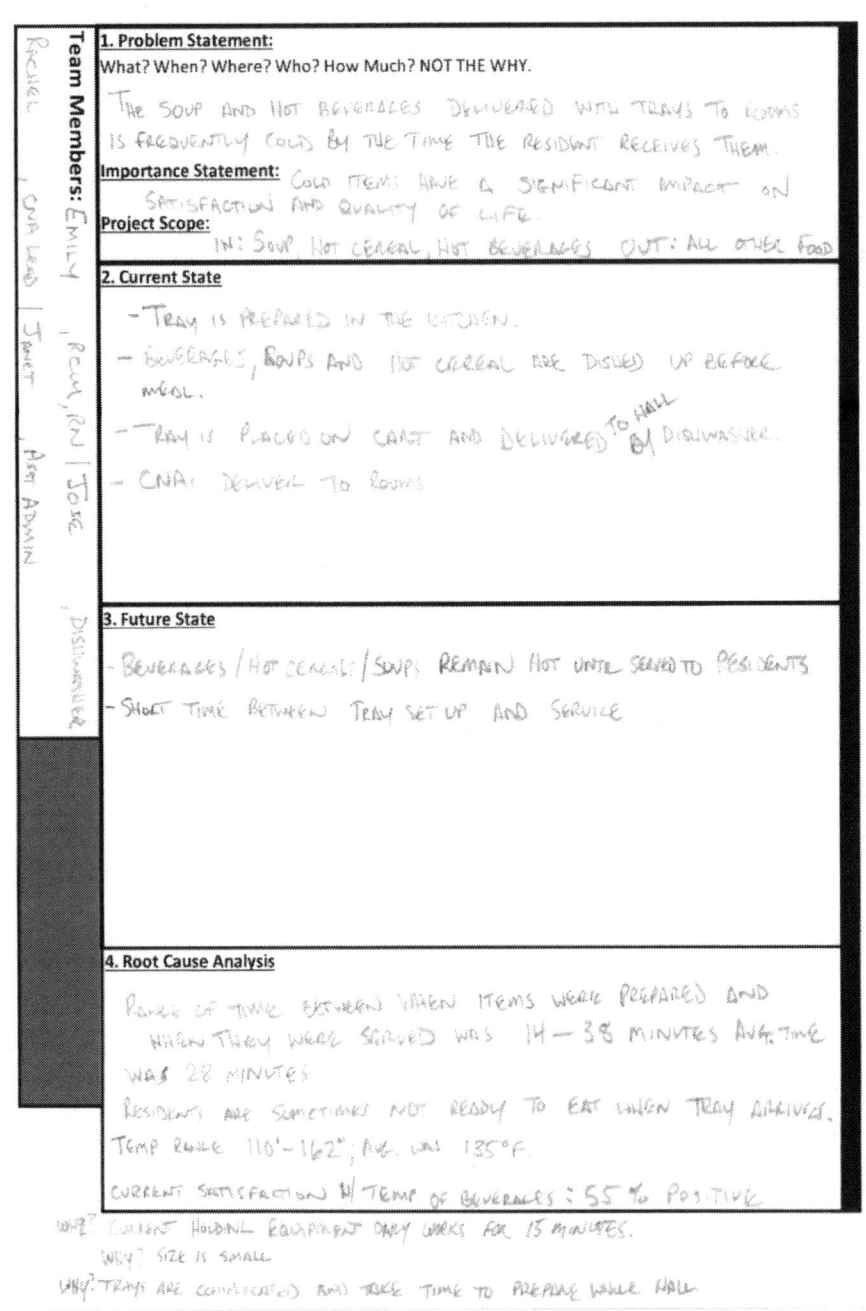

Example of an A3 Document exploring beverage temperatures (left side)

5. Solutions/ Countermeasures

Gap No.	Countermeasure (If we…)	Outcome (Then we should get…)	Metric
1.	Hot beverages poured into carafes and delivered to halls. Soup/hot cereal put in tureen and delivered to halls.	Beverages should be hot at service	Temp

6. Testing and Pilot Projects

Experiment	Anticipated Effect	Actual Effect
Test use of carafes & tureens on Bridgeview Hall	Food/beverage temp ↑	Coffee avg temp: 172° Tea avg temp: 179° Soup avg temp: 162°

7. Completion Plan

What?	Who?	When?
Expand to other halls	Emily, RCM Laurie, RCM	August 15

8. Confirmed State:

GARDENVIEW:
COFFEE TEMP: RANGE 171-175° AVG 174°
SOUP TEMP: RANGE 160-170° AVG 165°

CHESTNUT:
COFFEE - R 169°-177° AVG 174°
OATMEAL - R 172°-185° AVG 178°

HAZELTON:
COFFEE - R 170°-177° AVG 175°
SOUP - R 159°-170° AVG 166°

SATISFACTION W/ TEMP OF BEVERAGES: 93% POSITIVE

9. Insights

+	Δ
Bridgeview did excellent job with pilot. Dining supplier helpful in brainstorming ideas	Ensure delivery of items before scheduling test - had to delay 1 wk and this caused confusion

How can we share these lessons and apply the learning elsewhere?

Begin exploring family style dining on halls.

* Still need more work to optimize tray line.

Example of an A3 Document exploring beverage temperatures (right side)

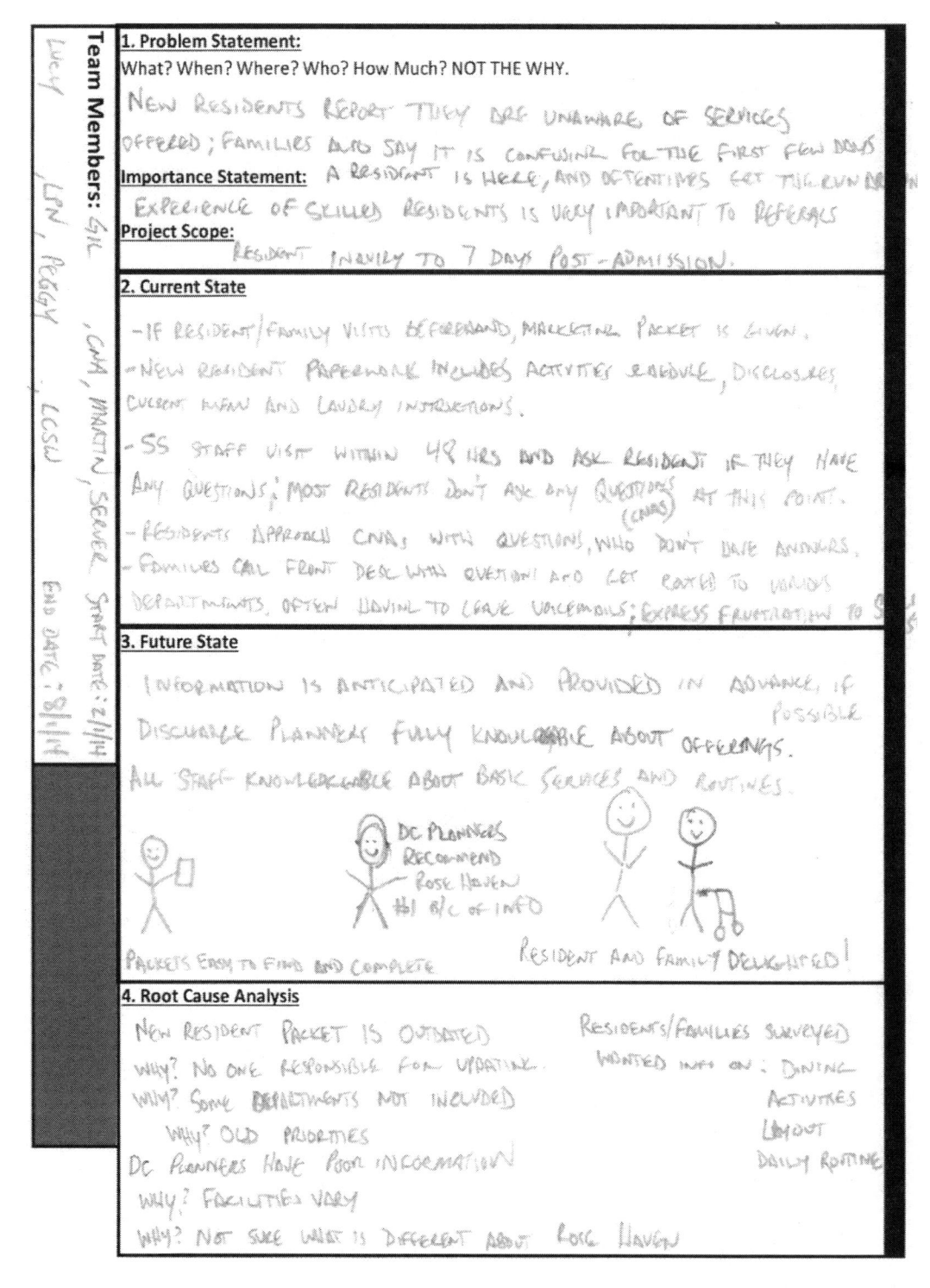

Team Members: Gil, CNA, Martin, Seeker, Lin, Peggy, Lucy, LCSW

Start Date: 2/1/14
End Date: 3/1/14

1. Problem Statement:
What? When? Where? Who? How Much? NOT THE WHY.

New residents report they are unaware of services offered; families also say it is confusing for the first few days.

Importance Statement: A resident is here, and oftentimes get the run down. Experience of skilled residents is very important to referrals.

Project Scope: Resident inquiry to 7 days post-admission.

2. Current State

- If resident/family visits beforehand, marketing packet is given.
- New resident paperwork includes activity schedule, disclosures, current menu and laundry instructions.
- SS staff visit within 48 hrs and ask resident if they have any questions; most residents don't ask any questions at this point.
- Residents approach CNAs with questions, who don't have answers. (CNAs)
- Families call front desk with questions and get routed to various departments, often having to leave voicemails; express frustration to SS

3. Future State

Information is anticipated and provided in advance, if possible.
Discharge planners fully knowledgeable about offerings.
All staff knowledgeable about basic services and routines.

DC Planners recommend Rose Haven #1 b/c of info

Packets easy to find and complete

Resident and family delighted!

4. Root Cause Analysis

New resident packet is outdated
Why? No one responsible for updating.
Why? Some departments not included
Why? Old priorities

DC Planners have poor information
Why? Facilities vary
Why? Not sure what is different about Rose Haven

Residents/Families surveyed wanted info on: Dining, Activities, Layout, Daily Routine

Example of an A3 Document exploring information for new residents (left side)

5. Solutions/ Countermeasures

Gap No.	Countermeasure (If we...)	Outcome (Then we should get...)	Metric
1	Revise new resident packet	Better, more relevant info	Satisfaction %
2	Develop materials for DC planners	Knowledgeable DC planners	Knowledge %

6. Testing and Pilot Projects

Experiment	Anticipated Effect	Actual Effect	
New packet provided to resident in month of May	Satisfied w/ info provided: 75%	90%	
Visit DC planners at Three Rivers and Kaiser Skyline	Knowledgeable about services: 85%	70%	← Lower than expected — need to rework materials

7. Completion Plan

What?	Who?	When?
Distribute updated guide	Betty Lou, DNS	April 2nd
Update admission procedure	Betty Lou, DNS	April 2nd
Re-write DC planner guide	Sarah S, SW	April 15th
Distribute & test 2nd DC planner guide	Sarah S and Peggy N, SW	May 1st

8. Confirmed State:

30 Day satisfied w/ info provided: 90%

60 Day satisfied w/ info provided: 93%

30 Day knowledgeable about services: 90%

90 Day satisfied w/ info provided: 95%

60 Day knowledgeable about services: 95%

9. Insights

+	Δ
Clarified new resident process. Less anxiety for new residents	Continue learning about what people want to know beforehand. Include more CNAs on project team

How can we share these lessons and apply the learning elsewhere?

Need to review other handbooks and guides given to residents.

Example of an A3 Document exploring information for new residents (right side)

Team Members:

1. Problem Statement:
What? When? Where? Who? How Much? NOT THE WHY.

Importance Statement:

Project Scope:

2. Current State

3. Future State

4. Root Cause Analysis

5. Solutions/ Countermeasures

Gap No.	Countermeasure (If we…)	Outcome (Then we should get…)	Metric

6. Testing and Pilot Projects

Experiment	Anticipated Effect	Actual Effect

7. Completion Plan

What?	Who?	When?

8. Confirmed State:

9. Insights

+	Δ

How can we share these lessons and apply the learning elsewhere?

VALUE AND NON-VALUE ADDED WORK

IS WORK ADDING VALUE?

1. Are we providing or changing something?
- Item
- Service
- Experience

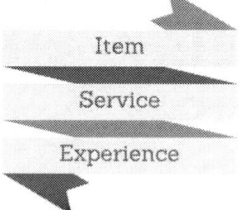

2. Is this something the customer wants?

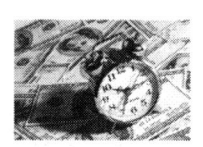

And is willing to pay with time or money?

3. Is it done right the first time?

Error-free, on-time

In Lean, we focus on creating value for residents. Value added work has three components:

1. **Something is changed or provided in a process.** This piece is pretty self-explanatory; to add value, we must do something. In typical aging services communities, this includes a range of things, from items (supplies, food, utilities), to services (healthcare, dining rooms, recreation and leisure), to experiences (life-care, aging-in-place, community).

This also applies to internal customers. For instance, the facilities team might be responsible for painting healthcare areas, dining may provide employee meals, and many departments may be responsible for forwarding service and supply usage to the billing office.

2. **Something that a customer (resident or internal customer) is willing to pay extra for, either in money, time or another resource.** This piece is key because it demonstrates that value is determined by the customer. We can (and do) put a lot of time and work into many things that residents don't necessarily want, but that doesn't add value. In addition, waiting time is almost always non-value added.

Similarly, we oftentimes have bureaucratic processes for internal customers—certain forms that must be completed a certain way or provide information that isn't really needed— these create work, but don't add value.

How do we know what someone wants (and is willing to pay for)? The easiest way is to ask. Collecting feedback from residents and staff is crucial to determining what work is adding value and what work isn't.

3. **Something that is done right the first time.** Mistakes or errors that we have to fix take an enormous amount of time and resources in most organizations. In many cases, investigations following errors aren't complete or don't address root causes, but still take up significant time with research and documentation. Indeed, some places operate almost continuously in a vicious cycle of making mistakes and then trying to correct them.

By focusing on these three, key components of value added work, we can break down all activities into what's important to residents and what isn't. The part of work that isn't valuable (non-value added), is generally waste (from the resident's perspective), and our goal is to eliminate as much of it as possible. (We'll dive deeper into waste a little later.)

As you are looking over the criteria of value added work, you can probably think of a number of things that don't fit into all three categories, but are nevertheless important: parts of the MDS assessment, some clinical documentation, and other activities that are required by regulation or standards of care. We call this work "non-value added, but necessary," and while we can never eliminate this sort of work, we can look for ways to minimize the time and resources we spend on it. By doing so, we focus our efforts on the work that matters most to residents.

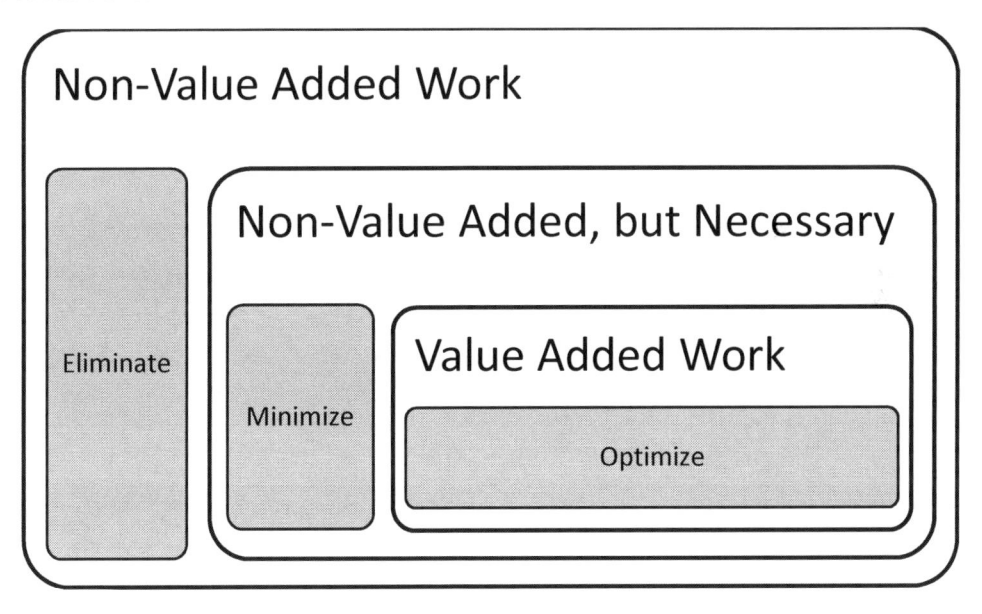

Non-Value Added Work
 Non-Value Added, but Necessary
  Value Added Work
   Optimize
  Minimize
 Eliminate

A great example of minimizing required work is charting by exception. Rather than charting irrelevant information, routine activities, or that nothing happened at all during a shift or day, focus charting on unusual or abnormal occurrences and information. In addition to saving the waste of extra charting, it reduces the time it takes to gather necessary information from the resident record and thus future waste.

Another area to examine for non-value added, but necessary work surrounds regulatory compliance and survey preparation. The regulatory burden on providers, especially nursing homes, is significant, but staff and administrators also sometimes establish excessive systems or do far more work that required "just to be safe." Instead of just accepting the extra work, reach out to regulators and surveyors to better understand requirements. Utilize provider trade organizations and other advocacy groups, as well. Creating better value in healthcare is a top national priority, with support from both the Centers for Medicare and Medicaid and state-based agencies, so there is likely to be increasing support for reducing unnecessary compliance work.

Lean is not a good strategy to find ways to eliminate staff. If people fear their jobs will be cut, they will not actively engage in improvement work. What you will find in adopting Lean, however, is a lot of waste due to departmental silos. It's natural (and good) to see some departments shrink and others grow as a result of optimizing processes. Provide staff with opportunities to learn different skills and transfer departments as necessary. Adaptability and flexibility are key requirements in organizations that succeed with Lean, and you should not discount the need to spend time addressing the personal concerns of staff during improvement activities, including the fear of changing job duties and the loss of no longer doing work they may have done for many years.

A final note: people are NEVER non-value added. It's always important to show respect for people doing work, even if the work itself doesn't add value. As waste is removed from a process, staff need to be supported in the transition to value-added work.

Value added activities	Non-value added, but necessary activities	Non-value added activities
• Personal care support • Desireable leisure activities • Food that a resident prefers • Therapy that helps a resident maintain or improve • Safe home environment	• MDS sections that don't improve care provided to a resident • Incident investigations and reports • Some recordkeeping and required audits • Insurance-required documentation	• Poor care • Unwanted food items • Time spent searching for supplies, equipment • Audits and quality checks not required by regulation • Work done "just in case"

WASTE

No one likes waste. When we see something we think is wasteful, we usually try to correct it. In resource-scarce environments, like most nursing homes and other communities, waste is particularly scorned because there are rarely enough resources for even what's necessary. Unfortunately, waste isn't always easy to see. Extra food thrown out after a meal is easy to identify, but what about the food left on a resident's plate? It's just as much waste as food thrown away in the kitchen. Extra checking and oversight because we don't trust staff to do their jobs is also wasteful. Waiting and walking around because there isn't enough equipment or supplies available where they are needed happens surprisingly often, and represents another manifestation of waste.

Waste is bad in and of itself. But more so, it oftentimes represents something else: hidden problems— defects, slow processes, extra walking, and unnecessary oversight. Waste creeps in over time when we aren't aware or paying attention. Gloves run out, so staff begin keeping a stockpile hidden. A medication reconciliation process isn't followed correctly, so an audit and layer of oversight is added. Waste allows problems to be ignored, covered up, or repaired so that a process can be completed. Instead of adding wasteful activities, however, we should spend the time to identify the root cause of a problem and address that instead, removing the need to add wasteful work or extra process steps.

Waste is work that isn't wanted or needed, and it causes resources—money and time—to be diverted away from caring for residents. Searching for waste identifies underlying problems that need to be addressed, which then allows us to better serve residents. Learning to see waste takes time—indeed, much waste is simply absorbed into our daily routines so much that we don't notice—but once you start, you'll be amazed at how much you find.

As noted earlier, many forms of waste in aging services are further hidden by our current payment models, especially fee-for-service and per diem models. Many care mistakes, for instance, don't have direct or certain costs. These models are quickly changing, however, and organizations that can hone their focus on value will reap large benefits under value-based payment programs. In addition, value is intimately tied to satisfaction, and if you want to be successful marketing to the next wave of residents and their families, hospitality and satisfaction should be only slightly second to quality of care.

We can categorize waste into eight different types and remember them with the acronym DOWNTIME: Defects, Overproduction, Waiting, Non-Utilized Talent, Transportation, Inventory, Motion, and Excess Processing.

Defects

Defects are errors or mistakes. Defects cause duplication of efforts, as work must be redone, and sometimes lead to even more work if the mistake causes an adverse outcome or incident. Examples of defects:

- Failing to document care
- Improper cleaning of a catheter
- Preparing a meal tray with the wrong diet order
- Adverse drug reactions and medication errors
- Outdated or inaccurate care plans
- Preventable nosocomial infections

Defects in care and services are unfortunately frequent, yet usually hidden. Many times, care mistakes aren't even known unless they lead to an adverse outcome. The key is to create a culture where staff learn to recognize *all mistakes* so that root causes can be identified and addressed.

In addition to the waste of actual errors, consider also the waste of error inspection and detection activities. For those who are steeped in the culture of long-term care, inspection and oversight activities seem almost second nature. Indeed, a typical response to any sort of problem or error is to create an audit or oversight mechanism, whereby a manager reviews a process or outcome to ensure it is free of errors. But in an ideal world, where work is done correctly the first time, inspection and oversight activities are just another form of waste. While some of these review processes may be required by regulation, it is useful to carefully examine how to minimize the non-value added portions. Inspection and detection wastes includes:

- Quality assurance review and utilization review committees
- Chart audits
- Legal and risk management inspections

Overproduction

Overproduction is making more of something than is needed. The most visible kind of overproduction typically occurs in ancillary services, such as dining and facilities management. Examples include:

- Preparing food in large batches that goes unused
- Setting up more tables or chairs than an event needs
- Making too many copies of a form that will soon be updated

Another type of overproduction common in healthcare is when parallel structures do the same thing. This is when two different people (or two different departments/ facilities/ etc.)

complete the same work independent of each other. Oftentimes, these structures are created due to silos between departments or facilities, or, increasingly, when a community adopts a new technology (like an Electronic Health Record, care pathways tool, new call system) that attempts to streamline work. In cases of the latter, it is very important to revise your old workflows to take advantage of the new technology and ensure you aren't just doing more work. Some examples of overproduction due to parallel structures are:

- Keeping duplicate personnel files in HR and home departments
- Information stored in an Electronic Health Record and in separate Excel files (or still on paper)
- Redundant recordkeeping due to oversight or quality control
- Individual procedures for the same work in different departments or different communities
- Improving programs or processes in multiple departments without sharing learnings and best practices between them

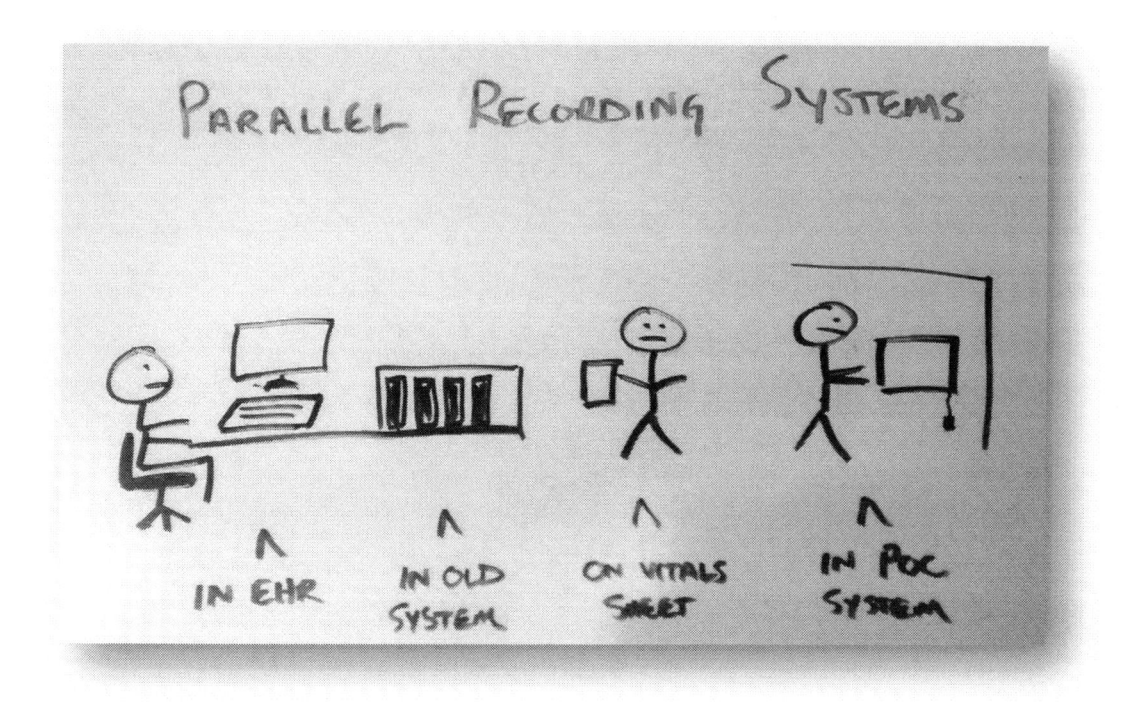

Several years after a CCRC had implemented an Electronic Medical Record, a review of their bowel monitoring program revealed that staff were inputting the same data in four different places. This is a common occurrence when implementing technology solutions likes EMRs.

Waiting

Waiting is both an obvious waste and an invisible one. We know that waiting is a large part of most processes in our work, but we also become blind to how long staff and residents spend waiting every single day. Sometimes it's hidden in other wastes, too (such as walking back and forth to check if something is ready). Waiting also leads to multi-tasking, which causes small amounts of waste between each changeover of activities. Examples of waiting might be:

- Residents waiting for an aide to be available for personal care
- Staff and resident waiting for a lift to be available
- When a nurse is needed to perform a resident assessment before another action can occur
- Approvals that require an administrator to sign off on
- Submitting orders to medical records and waiting for new MARs or TARs to be printed
- When staff aren't available to transport a resident to an activity or mealtime

Non-Utilized Talent

Non-utilized talent includes restrictive policies and procedures that don't allow employees to complete work they otherwise are capable of, burdening staff with more work than is reasonable (leading to fatigue and poor engagement), and other environmental factors that inhibit employee participation. Organizational structure, such as burdensome or antagonistic personnel policies, and work cultures that support a top-down management approach, also contribute to non-utilized talent. Consider the following:

- Policies that limit who can enter resident rooms or other work areas (such as kitchens)
- Policies that restrict the scope of practice unnecessarily
- Inconsistent application of workplace practices
- Blaming employees for system errors
- Practices that restrict decision-making authority
- Stressful or harsh work environments that cause employees to disengage or not participate in improvement activities

Transportation

Transportation is unnecessary movement in processes, generally related to having to move residents or supplies. Transportation waste occurs in the following examples:

- Moving residents to a central space for activities, dining, etc.
- Storage areas far from staff work areas
- Long hallways and corridors
- Moving equipment back and forth between neighborhoods

Inventory

Extra supplies cost resources and take up valuable space. While certainly long-term care communities need to maintain supplies to prevent outages, excess inventory leads to clutter and is frequently an inefficient use of money. Additionally, many supplies expire if they are not used quickly enough, leading to the total loss of the product. Some examples of inventory waste are:

- Medication supplies in excess of what can be used in a timely fashion
- Overcrowded central supply rooms
- Hidden stashes of gloves, incontinent products, washcloths, etc.
- Food products that aren't used before spoilage

Motion

Motion is waste related to staff movement. Movement waste can lead to employee injuries and interrupts the flow of work. Examples of motion waste include:

- Room set ups that require excessive bending and twisting when completing tasks
- Shower/ spa rooms designed without ready access to soap, shampoo, towels, etc.
- Tray lines not optimized for movement
- Walking to another neighborhood to retrieve a lift
- Walking to another work area to check if a process is done or a resident is ready

Excess Processing

Excess processing is doing more work than is required. This may seem silly, but it is actually one of the more common forms of waste found in aging services. Excess processing takes many forms:

- Charting beyond what is needed
- Extra quality checks or oversight because of past problems or unreliable processes
- Communicating more than what is needed, or more often than is needed
- Writing memos that aren't read
- Creating and filling out forms that don't serve a useful purpose
- Centralizing decision-making for trivial matters (i.e., Management needs to approve any small decision, regardless of the impact)

CONFUSION

In her book A3 Problem Solving for Healthcare, Cindy Jimmerman makes the argument that confusion can be considered a primary waste in healthcare. (Jimmerman, 2007, p. 8) Certainly, anyone who has spent time in any segment of healthcare can relate to the confusion sometimes present.

In long-term care communities, confusion appears in many forms and places: unclear care plans, outdated notes posted in work areas, unclear responsibilities, differing assumptions by management and line staff, unworkable policies and procedures that require staff to invent their own processes—the list could go on. In many cases, there are other wastes either causing or being caused by confusion, so it's useful to examine carefully the situation causing confusion. As a first step, it's important to take staff concerns about confusion at face value. All too often, managers and administrators will assume that staff should know what to do, either because it's "obvious," "they've been told a hundred times," or "the policy and procedure is crystal clear." This type of thinking inevitable leads to a constant cycle of fire-fighting, responding to problems, disciplinary action, and turnover. To break this constant cycle, investigate circumstances when someone is unclear or confused about work. Ask about the specific sources of confusion, drilling down to root causes and addressing them.

IDENTIFYING WASTE

Learning to see waste takes time and practice. Taiichi Ohno, the early Lean pioneer at Toyota, used to draw a small chalk circle on the shop floor and have new managers stand there until they had identified all of the waste in that work area. A modern approach is called the 30-30-30 exercise. (Protzman, Mayzell, & Kerpchar, 2011, pp. 88-90) Spend 30 minutes in a work area trying to identify at least 30 instances of waste. Then spend 30 minutes on reducing just one. In just an hour, you'll probably be amazed at how much you can learn.

Outside eyes can be very helpful in identifying waste. Talk to your vendors and delivery drivers about your goals to identify waste. (Be sure to offer a little explanation on what you mean by "waste.") Vendors see and hear a lot of things in the back corridors of your buildings, and their input can be invaluable. Another great source is to assign the 30-30-30 exercise above to an entire leadership team, but have each manager spend time in a work area other than the one they oversee.

It's not uncommon for people to become defensive when someone from outside of their department or building offers observations or insights. This is normal, and demonstrates the pride and ownership of work that staff have. It's important, though, to remember the goal of Lean is to continuously improve work. Be cautious about "sacred cows" or areas and people that are off-limits to criticism; waste is present in everyone's work area. Develop strong team support around waste reduction as a way to better serve residents. No matter what the explanation for the waste is, embrace the feedback, thank the sharer for providing it, and work to eliminate it.

Waste Identification Audit

	Details/ Picture of Waste
Defects Errors and mistakes, efforts spent to review and fix errors and mistakes	
Overproduction Making more of something than can be used	
Waiting Non-productive use of time due to lack of people, equipment or materials	
Non-Utilized Talent Skill, talent, or ability not being used to fullest potential	
Transportation Unnecessary movement of people or materials	
Inventory Materials and supplies purchased but not immediately used	
Motion Unnecessary movement of employees within a work area	
Extra Processing Doing more work on a process than is required by the resident or other customer	

STANDARDIZED WORK

One of the most common problems in long-term care involves line staff not following correct work procedures. Why is this? Long-term care communities have no shortage of policies and procedures, nor are they typically shy in disseminating them to staff over and over (usually after a disciplinary counseling or adverse event). Administrators and nursing managers spend countless hours a week reviewing the proper way to transfer a resident, clean a leg bag, or allow dishes to dry. Unfortunately, problems with compliance seem to reoccur, and significant time is spent fighting fires as a result.

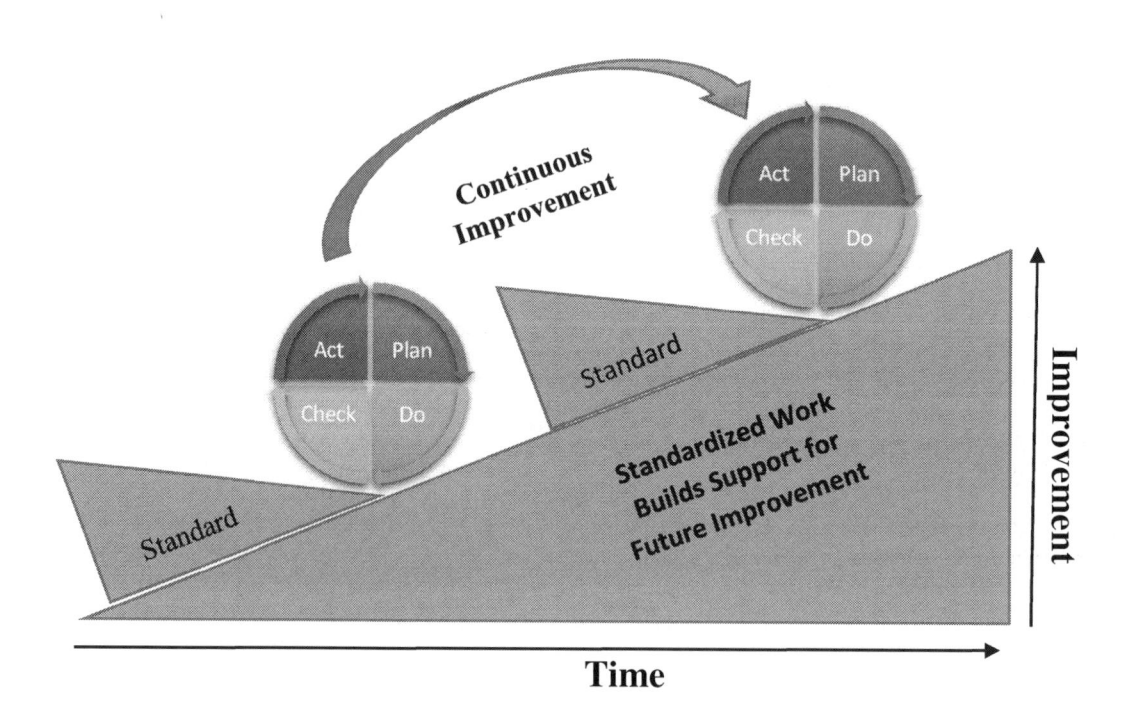

Lean uses a concept called standardized work to describe a more sustainable approach to process and work management. Standardized work is very different than a policy and procedure, and it creates a much different result, as well.

1) **Standardized work is written by those who do it.** You can't create standardized work in your office, nor can you create standardized work alone. Typically, the biggest obstacle is sitting in the office and trying to write out what staff are supposed to do. This is a recipe for disaster, and leads to policies and procedures that aren't practical, reasonable, or possible with the time and equipment available.

43

Standardized work is accomplished by having those who do the work write out the process. Managers need to be involved too, particularly making sure all regulatory requirements are addressed, but line staff should lead the exercise. In doing so, leaders often learn of hidden problems and reasons why work changes over time. This provides a great opportunity to engage in problem solving work, helping the team to overcome challenges while meeting any regulatory or corporate needs.

2) **Standardized work is the best knowledge at the time and must be changed whenever improvements occur.** Policies and procedures (P&P's) tend to last far longer than their usefulness, and it's not uncommon to find P&Ps that haven't been reviewed or updated for years. In addition, line staff typically view P&Ps as mandates from above that must be followed regardless of whether they make sense or describe the best way to accomplish work. Standardized work, on the other hand, is designed to be changed as needed to reflect the best practice at the time. By tasking them with the primary responsibility to write the process, line staff are more likely to feel empowered to change the work as they discover better ways to accomplish tasks.

3) **Standardized work must be clearly displayed.** Standardized work serves as both a guide for line staff and a tool for supervisors to ensure work processes are completed corrected. By communicating the information clearly, and placing the information in easily accessible places (NOT in a binder on the shelf that no one reads!), it's much easier for employees to do what is expected of them.

4) **Standardized work makes orientation much more effective and complete.** How many times have you hired a new staff person only to find they are trained "the wrong way" by their trainer? With turnover between 30% and 75% in most communities, consistency of training is a huge concern. Standardized work helps ensure consistency because it represents the best way to accomplish a task. It also provides an easy to understand, easy to follow guide to the work expected of new staff.

5) **When standardized work is not being followed, managers must ask why.** In typical environments, managers respond to failure to follow work procedures by admonishing or disciplining an employee and requiring compliance. Lean requires a different approach. Instead, managers must ask the employee why the standardized work is not being followed. Employees rarely choose to do bad work for the sake of doing bad work. Instead, other problems (the root causes) such as not having adequate equipment or supplies, not having enough time, or an outdated practice are the reasons behind deviation. By asking why and finding the actual problems, we help to create better work environments for all staff, leading to better care and service to residents.

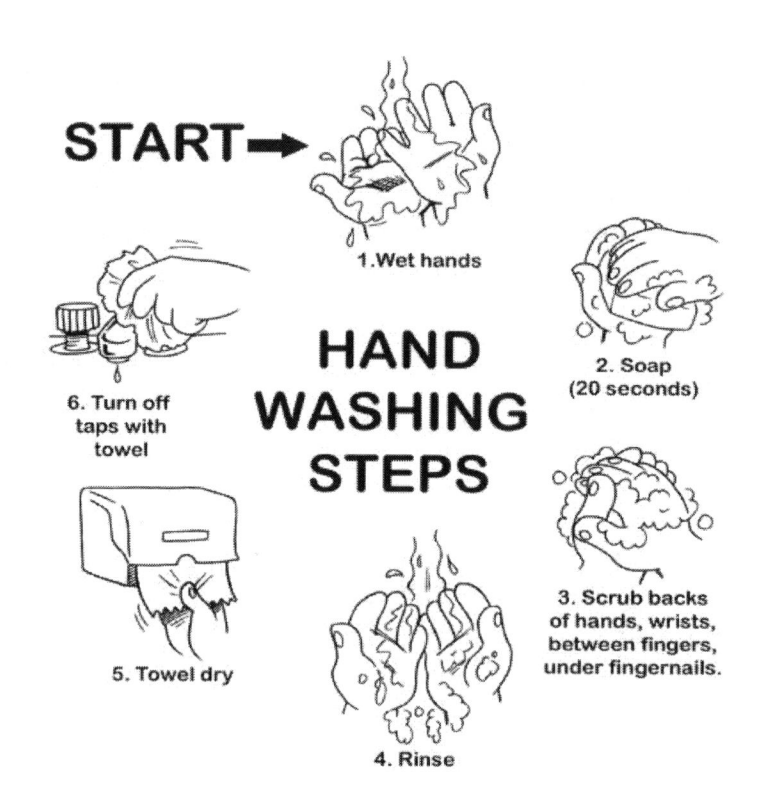

Example of handwashing standard work

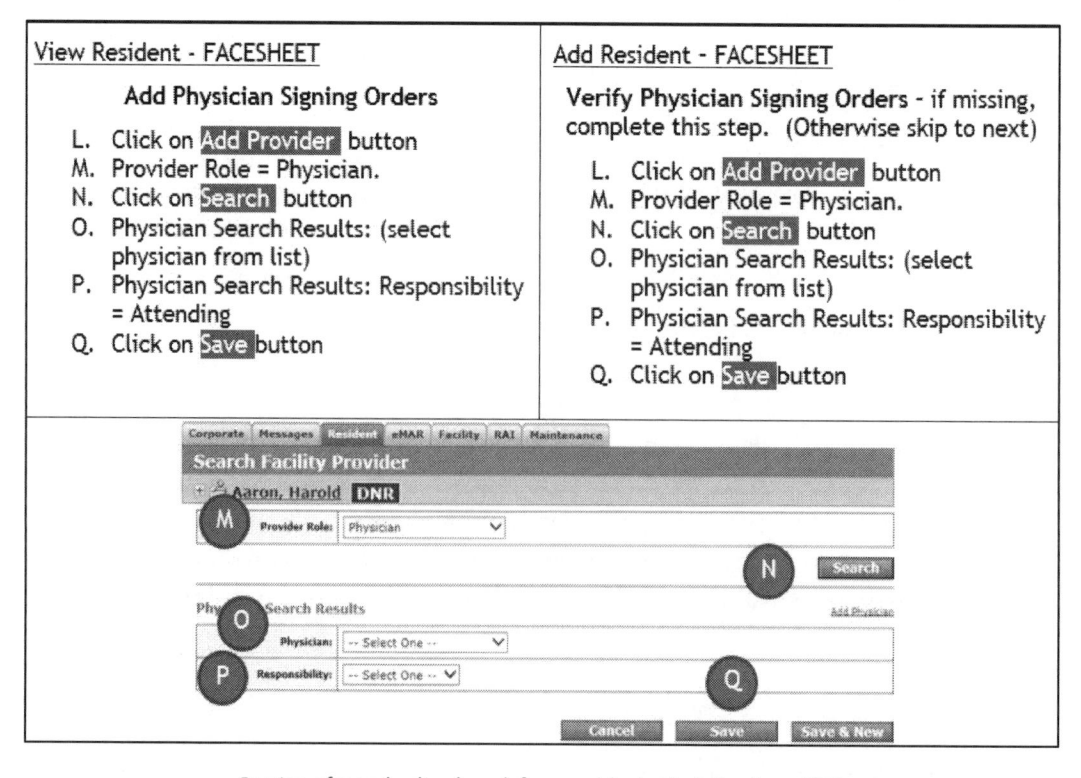

View Resident - FACESHEET	Add Resident - FACESHEET
Add Physician Signing Orders L. Click on Add Provider button M. Provider Role = Physician. N. Click on Search button O. Physician Search Results: (select physician from list) P. Physician Search Results: Responsibility = Attending Q. Click on Save button	**Verify Physician Signing Orders** - if missing, complete this step. (Otherwise skip to next) L. Click on Add Provider button M. Provider Role = Physician. N. Click on Search button O. Physician Search Results: (select physician from list) P. Physician Search Results: Responsibility = Attending Q. Click on Save button

Portion of standardized work for a resident admission in an EHR

LEADER STANDARDIZED WORK

Standardized work is not only designed to guide line staff; it works equally well—and is equally important—for leaders, too. Standardized work for leaders consists of developing routines for rounding with purpose (going to the gemba) and other activities where you check in on the status of current tactical and strategic goals.

A purposeful, daily stand-up meeting is a good start to standardized work. It should consist of sharing census changes, resident concerns, staffing issues, safety incidents, future events and successes to be celebrated. Once you have started building a culture of continuous improvement, consider adding a minute of reflection. Ask the team, "How did yesterday go?" and "What can we do better today?" The idea of building upon each day keeps work from being routine and helps staff to engage in the process of making small improvements all the time. A stand-up meeting should start on time consistently and last no more than 10 or 15 minutes. For issues that require more than a minute or two of discussion, have a smaller group break off afterwards to discuss rather than occupying everyone's time.

Developing a daily checklist that incorporates current goals is another way to standardize oversight and accountability. A daily checklist helps to reinforce priorities, communicate the intended direction of the organization, and connect to the drivers that will lead to the desired goals. The questions need to be customized to your current goals and priorities to be effective. Generally, improving resident quality and experience are top concerns of most organizations, as are employee staffing and performance issues. If there is significant construction, reorganization or major initiatives rolling out, these items should be integrated into the daily checklist.

Sometimes, questions may seem formulaic or unnatural. Don't worry. If staff know that they can count on a response, they will be happy to share struggles and challenges. Also, by asking questions like, "Have there been any falls in the last 24 hours?" or "Are all assessments up to date?" staff will understand the importance of these items to your work and to the organization's overall success. Questions should change over time as priorities and goals do.

For non-daily, but regular activities, it's a good idea to schedule them on your calendar so they occur. Just as most organizations have regularly scheduled committee and department meetings, you should have scheduled mentoring meetings with key employees, check-ins with department managers, and time allotted to review team improvement projects, both that are in progress and have been completed.

Mentoring employees should be a large part of a leader's standardized work. In traditional environments, leaders were responsible (and expected) to solve most problems. As you have probably gathered by now, Lean takes a much different approach. Every employee must be part of the problem solving team, and the primary role of leaders is not to provide solutions, but rather provide support, teaching, and access to needed resources. As you make the transition to empowered teams, some supervisors and department managers will fit in perfectly. Indeed, they have probably long practiced team-based learning and problem solving.

Others—especially those who have been very successful leaders in the past—may struggle with mentoring their line staff. Instead of pushing their team to grow, they may continue to control most of the problem solving process themselves, doling out solutions and fixing errors through their own work and oversight of the process. Sometimes this comes from a belief that staff are too busy to fix problems. (And sometimes they are—but this is a problem to address separately!) Other times, leaders believe that line staff can't be trusted or relied upon to do accurate and thorough work, so how could they possibly be involved in making the situation better?

This is why it is imperative that you regularly check in with front-line leaders to learn not only what problems staff are having, but also to observe how teams are going about resolving those problems. Are they using the A3 and PDSA process? Are line staff actively engaged in the work? Is the leader providing more support and training than answers and oversight? If you discover that the leader is having trouble engaging and mentoring their staff, find out the root cause and address it with the leader. If the problem is trust-based, look at how to develop better communication and accountability systems within that team. If the issue is related to the leader feeling like his or her team doesn't have enough time to participate in problem solving, figure out ways to work together to free up staff time. (This might be a great opportunity to spend some time in the *gemba* yourself by covering some line duties for a short period on a regular basis until the process gets going.)

Administrator Daily Check Sheet

Week Of: _____

Question	M	T	W	R	F	Weekly Notes
Have there been any resident incidents in the last 24 hours?						Mon
Any resident complaints/ concerns in the last 24 hours?						
Any census concerns or insurance challenges?						
Any vendor concerns or challenges?						Tue
Have there been any employee injuries or accidents in the last 24 hours?						
Are any employees on light-duty or off due to injury?						
Are there any employee staffing issues?						Wed
Are there any employee performance issues?						
Any significant personal issues affecting a staff member?						
Are there any supply or equipment problems?						Thur
Any performance projects experiencing difficulty or need extra support?						
Are there any barriers I can remove?						
Is there anyone who should be recognized for outstanding work?						Fri
Nursing						
Are incident trends in line with expectations?						
Any training needs to consider?						**Reminders for Next Week**
Building Services						
Any physical plant concerns?						
Any budget concerns?						
Dining						
Any food or labor cost concerns or trends?						
What are current top resident concerns?						
Activities						
What upcoming events should I be aware of?						
Any inter-department challenges or successes I should know?						
Social Work						
Any complaint/ concern trends?						
Anticipated admissions/discharges for the next week?						

DON Daily Check Sheet   Week Of: _____

Question	M	T	W	R	F	Weekly Notes
Have there been any resident incidents in the last 24 hours?						Mon
How many resident falls in the last 24 hours?						
Have there been any unusual resident complaints/ concerns in the last 24 hours?						Tue
Are all assessments currently up to date?						
Are there any current issues with Dr.'s, Clinics, Etc?						
Have there been any employee injuries or accidents in the last 24 hours?						Wed
Are any employees on light-duty or off due to injury?						
Are there any employee staffing issues?						
Are there any employee performance issues?						Thur
Any significant personal issues affecting a staff member?						
Are there any supply or equipment problems?						
Are there any barriers I can remove?						Fri
Is there anyone who should be recognized for outstanding work?						
Is there anything I can help with?						**Reminders for Next Week**

VISUAL CONTROLS

A highly visible workplace makes it much easier to know what to do and how to do it. Most visual control in aging services, however, takes the form of hastily written and poorly worded signs hung anywhere and everywhere. "Wash your hands!" "Label and date food!" "CLEAN UP AFTER YOURE SELF!!!!!111"

> It is every nurse's responsibilities to make sure all residents are getting the correct meds. This is basic nursing. There is no excuse for med errors. It is your nurse's license that you are risking. If you are missing any medication **DO NOT BORROW.** It is your responsibility to call pharmacy and get that med delivered, if for any reason it will not be here when it is scheduled, **YOU** need to call the Dr. and get an order to hold or give at a later time. Every one of you should read and re-read the regulations for a correct med pass which you have been inserviced and trained. As I'm sure everyone knows we received a state tag from IDPH regarding failure to comply with the rules and regulations of med pass. Everyone one of you has been in-serviced on how to do a correct med pass and are now being audited. Now is the time to ask questions. You should be doing this correctly every day so it's no surprise when you are being audited. When IDPH returns they **WILL** be watching you pass meds. If there are any errors you will likely be listed on their "E" key by name. This can be detrimental not only to the facility's license, but also to yours. Moving forward progressive disciplinary action up to and possibly including termination, will be taken for failure to comply with the rules and regulations of med pass. If you feel you need additional training, it is your responsibility to request such.

A note left at a nursing station. The length, poor grammar, and accusatory tone will likely cause it to have very little impact on staff behavior. It may also lead to resentment and anger.

A visual workplace is "self-ordering, self-explaining, self-regulating, and self-improving—where what is supposed to happen does happen, on time, every time, because of visual solutions." (Galsworth, 2005, p. 31) Effective visual controls provide guidance to employees and residents. They remove ambiguity and eliminate questions about what to do and where things should go. For example, taping the floor of areas that need to remain clear or where specific carts should be placed; easy-to-read, color-coded labels in storerooms; pictures along with words for work procedures.

Consider these examples:

The top note is accusatory and just lines of text. After a day or two, staff probably won't even notice it.

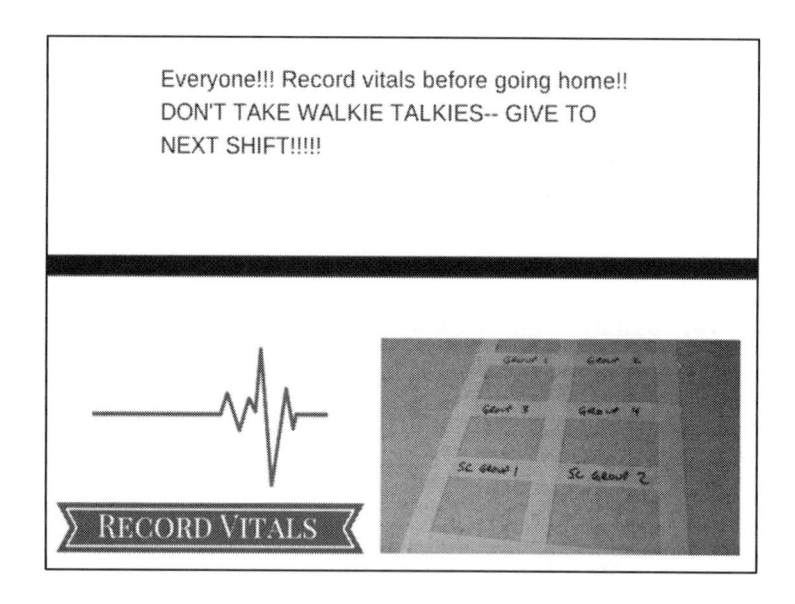

In contrast, the "record vitals" sign has a visual heartbeat to make the meaning clearer. On the right, taped locations on a desk help staff to remember where to put their walkie-talkie and make it easier to identify if any are missing before the staff member heads home.

Storerooms and equipment areas should be well-labeled and organized in a logical or useful fashion. Use colors, shapes, and example pieces to aide in quick identification of items.

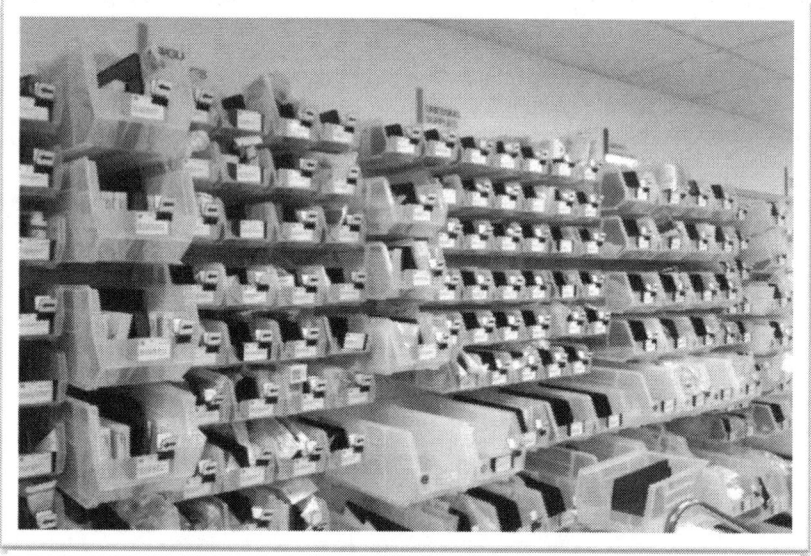

Color coded tags and box sizes, along with clear signage, helps staff quickly locate items in this storeroom

If you have identified a change while caring for or observing a resident, please **circle** the change and notify a nurse. Either give th nurse a copy of this tool or review it with her/him as soon as you can

S Seems different than usual
T Talks or communicates less
O Overall needs more help
P Pain – new or worsening; Participated less in activities

a
n Ate less
d No bowel movement in 3 days; or diarrhea
Drank less

W Weight change
A Agitated or nervous more than usual

A part of the "Stop and Watch" tool from INTERACT III that uses a short acronym on a pocket card to remind staff of things that they should report to a nurse. (For the full card and other training materials, visit the INTERACT site: http://www.interact2.net

HUDDLES

Daily attention to challenges and goals is the best way to ensure the organization is making progress. Huddles are quick, daily meetings where staff review current performance and targets, communicate about problems or challenges, and seek support from colleagues and supervisors. Huddles can cascade, too; in a typically community, administrative, department heads and nursing supervisors might attend one huddle, while each department might have a separate huddle during each shift. Issues that cannot be resolved at lower-level huddles should be escalated to higher-level huddles for support and resourcing. By doing so, it is possible to scale huddles from the front line of an assisted living to a national main office, eliminating much of the oversight work of regional operations staff and area managers.

Many long-term care and skilled nursing communities have long utilized a daily stand-up meeting, though the focus typically is on census and MDS concerns and usually includes only department managers and administrators. If you currently have a daily meeting, use this as a framework for your huddle. For providers without a current daily meeting, adding one will help bring challenges to the forefront and aid in accomplishing goals and meeting targets.

To build an effective daily huddle, hold the meeting every day at the same time. It should be short and begin and end on time, lasting no more than 15 minutes. The content of the meeting depends on both the community setting and current challenges or goals, but this is a useful framework to help create an agenda:

1. What admissions/ move-ins, discharges/ move-outs, change of status/ payer/ condition do we expect?
2. Any resident incidents or injuries in the past 24 hours? If so, a give brief description of the event and the current plan of care.
3. Any employee injuries or near misses in the past 24 hours? If so, give a brief description and any interim interventions to prevent reoccurrence.
4. Review current quality goals and areas of focus. (This should be specific to the community, and relate to mid- and long-term quality improvement goals; e.g., a community working to reduce the number of residents on antipsychotic medications would report daily on medication usage and describe any challenges or successes.)
5. Is there anything or anyone we need to celebrate or recognize?

For department level huddles, the focus should be tailored to particular needs and areas of concern. In dining, daily huddles might include a review of the daily menu, special events or celebrations, and any diet order changes or resident concerns. If a long-term goal relates to food temperatures, the daily huddle might also include reporting on a measure of this goal. In facilities and housekeeping, the focus may be on current work order status, projects in progress, and upcoming resident moves.

THE GEMBA WALK: HOW TO LEAD WITH RESPECT

"Go see, ask why, show respect" is a foundational Lean principle attributed to Fujio Cho, Toyota Motor Corporation Chairman. (Shook, 2011) It describes the core work of going to the place where work happens—the resident room, the medication room, the kitchen, the central laundry—to understand what is actually happening in an organization. In Lean, this is called the *gemba walk*. (*Gemba* means "the actual place," and refers to the physical place where work occurs, i.e. "the floor.") Once there, the manager must question why things happen as they are, discuss how they might be improved, and explore why problems may be occurring. During this process, it is imperative that the manager is respectful of the work area, the expertise of the people involved in the work, and the people themselves. Remember, respect for people, and especially front-line staff, is key to success with Lean.

A *gemba* walk might seem similar to the "management by walking/ wandering around" practice sometimes advocated by leadership experts. While both activities occur in the place where employees do work, a *gemba* walk is very, very different. It is purposeful instead of random, and seeks to directly connect with the people and work rather than simply observe and be available.

Michael Ballé describes a model of seven practices of lead with respect: Challenge, Teach, Listen, Learn, Support, Teamwork, and Go and See. (Balle, 2014) Go and see is not simply about being physically present in the workplace; it involves very purposeful and transformational activities:

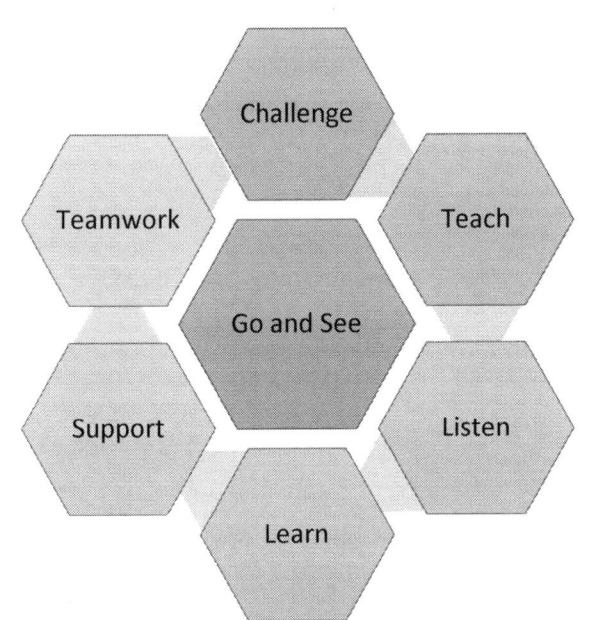

- **Challenge**: Press employees to think deeply and critically about issues. Encourage a culture of deep thinking and thorough understanding by pushing employees to problem solve rather than doing the work for them.
- **Teach**: Give staff the tools and training to engage in their work and address challenges that come up. When you discover that a staff member isn't aware of a procedure or doesn't know how to complete a task, take the opportunity to teach them the correct way. Consider that teaching is a very different concept than training. Training describes a process where information is given or provided, whereas teaching describes an interactive process where the recipient of information learns.

- **Listen**: Encourage ideas and feedback by listening and responding to staff. Listening involves both being quiet and hearing what the other person is saying as well as responding to let the other person know they were heard. Listening can also be quite difficult, especially when hearing something that is different than what you were expecting. When you are early on the Lean journey, it is crucial to be patient and open to feedback, even if it is uncomfortable to hear, as this will set the stage to building deeper trust with staff.
- **Learn**: Staff doing the everyday work are experts in what needs to be done and what challenges are getting in the way. Learn from their experience.
- **Support**: Sustain a culture of blame-free problem solving and provide adequate tools and training for employees to do their job without excessive stress or anxiety. If employees appear overworked, provide both immediate assistance in helping them complete their duties as well as longer-term support by investigating root causes.
- **Teamwork**: Enable staff to work together as a team. This means both establishing a culture of respect and communication and giving staff time and resources to meet regularly, discuss challenges, and create solutions. In addition, work hard to establish a sense of team between line staff and supervisory/management staff. Everyone's goal should be to serve the resident, and a strong, functional team requires everyone's participation.

GO SEE

Going to the place of work is easy. You leave the office and go to the action. Now what? Watch. Listen. When considering the work, look at purpose (why is the work happening?), process (what is happening?) and people (who is involved?). Is the work aligned with what residents expect? Are processes following designed specifications? Are people actively engaged in the work?

The place of work is a socio-technical system. That is, it is made up of people and tasks that combine to produce the results achieved. That's why it's crucial to understand both processes and people to determine how aligned to the purpose the work is.

You may wonder where you can find the time to go and see the work being done. After all, you are probably busy filling out reports, reviewing incident logs, responding to family questions and employee complaints, and a sundry of other crucial tasks. The short answer is right now. Most of the work currently consuming administrators and long term care leaders is retrospective analysis and oversight of work. Sometimes, whole days are spent just reviewing what has already happened and whole committees sit around debating why.

To start, just try spending 15 minutes a day watching work. You can even do small tasks to ease your way into the work areas of line staff—particularly if they aren't used to you being there. Review the MAR at the med cart, sit in the dining room and have lunch with residents, chop onions in the kitchen, mop a resident's floor, fold laundry. The key is to be present where the work occurs.

ASK WHY

When you go to the place of work, you will find things you don't understand or are different than you expect them to be. Resist the urge to correct the staff member or remind them of a particular policy or procedure. Instead, find out why the person is doing the work the way that they are. If a shortcut is being used, challenge the person to understand why the shortcut is used rather than resolving the underlying issue. By digging deep, you will see how small problems snowball into bigger ones through our natural tendency to quickly address issues in the course of work rather than study the problem and attempt to resolve the underlying causes.

In addition to (hopefully) many good things, you will likely see the following happen: staff running back and forth to find supplies; employees running into problems; residents unhappy about policies; equipment broken or used improperly; staff taking shortcuts. Employees may also ask you what to do when they encounter an issue. Resist the urge to solve their problem. Rather than take the issue back to your office to fix, or quickly implement your own solution (even if you "know" it to be correct), take the time to work through the process of problem solving with individuals and small teams.

When teaching staff, it's important to balance challenging with coaching. You want to push employees to think critically about issues, but you don't want them to become frustrated and disengage.

At the beginning of this process, staff will likely respond to many questions by saying, "We didn't know we could do that," especially if the community has history of authoritarian-style leadership. It can take some time, but once staff understand that they are trusted and able to solve problems and enact changes, most will never want to go back to the old way of doing things.

By providing support, empowering teams to learn about and improve their own work, and actively listening to challenges, you build a robust and capable workforce that looks forward to management presence rather than scurrying at the footsteps of the administrator.

SHOW RESPECT

Showing respect for staff cannot be overstated. Work in this field is extremely hard, both physically and emotionally, and it's important to constantly recognize the contributions each team member makes. When you are in someone's work area, be sure to introduce yourself and explain why you are there. No one wants to work while feeling like they are being judged.

Listen. Listen to what employees say and refrain from judgments or quick solutions. Lean teachers can oftentimes fix problems faster than individual employees, but they recognize that they can't be everywhere at all times. Thus, it's more crucial to develop problem-solving thinking in each person. Remember, Lean is about ordinary people working with extraordinary processes to get great results.

Finally, and once again, don't blame employees for doing work a certain way, even if it's wrong or against policy. Find out why they are doing it that way. Most people don't purposefully do the wrong thing. Asking why something is happening a certain way provides an opportunity to get at the heart of challenges and begin implementing sustainable improvements rather than temporary band-aids.

DIRECT-CARE STAFF IN CARE PLANNING

Another way to apply the "going to the *Gemba*" method of Lean is to invite direct care and other line staff to care/ service planning meetings. While many communities already use various methods to include the insights of those working directly with residents, the value of having CNAs, dining room servers and housekeepers actually present in planning meetings cannot be overstated. First, they provide direct accounts of resident concerns, needs, and wishes. They are also typically more insightful about crafting service and care needs since they work so close to the resident. Second, they can improve communication with the direct care team by sharing the care/ service plan directly, thereby helping to overcome staff resistance that oftentimes occurs when care planning staff are out of touch with actual resident needs.

To balance out time constraints, some communities designate a block of time (10 or 15 minutes) during the planning meeting for a CNA to attend. Spreading out meetings throughout the week, rather than focusing them all at one time can help, too. (This requires more flexibility from support and administrative staff, but can easily be accomplished. As an added benefit, most families appreciate a flexible care planning schedule, as it generally makes it easier for them to attend and participate in the process.) Another option to help include dining staff is to substitute a server for the dietician or food service manager. Most food-related concerns have very little to do with nutrition, anyways, and servers can be much more effective at helping to deal with resident complaints in the dining room.

The final benefit of having direct care staff at care/ service planning meetings is that it communicates to everyone that those staff are effective, trusted members of the service team. Residents and families who view them as such are more likely to bring problems or concerns to them directly rather than dumping them on management staff. This helps to reinforce problem-solving at the place closest to the resident or concern.

UNEVENNESS AND PROCESS LEVELING

Unevenness is a problem in factory environments because it leads to bottlenecks and waiting in the production line. In long-term care, and especially nursing homes, there has been a strong movement to move away from the "factory mindset" of delivering care. Instead, we want care to be provided when a resident wants it. So is the problem of unevenness something to worry about? In most cases, we don't have many practices of large batching, like in a factory, hospital, or lab, nor is a lot of work appointment-driven, as in a clinic. So we need to approach unevenness in the work in a slightly different way.

Many of the challenges with providing resident-centered care come from not having enough time or labor when the service is requested. Residents are woken up on a facility schedule so that morning care, breakfast, the AM medication pass and morning treatments can all be provided in an efficient way. When we move to a resident-centered model, it might seem to take more time, especially if we change between tasks or have to do more work, like cooking breakfast orders individually instead of in a batch. Generally speaking, it's not possible to add more labor, so we need to be creative to provide better service.

If you look carefully at the traditional model, however, you can see enormous waste hidden from view, along with strong dissatisfaction from the residents we serve. Uneven flow is clearly evident when you examine different job categories. CNAs, for instance, are very busy at the beginning of the day. But after meals, there is usually considerable downtime. Dishwashers may be rushed after a meal, but oftentimes have free time beforehand. Maintenance workers and housekeepers typically have more flexible workloads, but still experience periods of rushing and periods of calm. In addition, doing things in batches, like cooking large amounts of food, leads to overproduction, lower quality and more waste.

The key to providing better and more even service is to reduce barriers between different types of work and different staff roles. Moving to an open dining system is sometimes accomplished by implementing a concept of "all-hands dining," where all available staff assist in the dining room to provide quicker service. CNAs, then, can assist housekeepers in cleaning resident rooms during the CNA's slow time. The Universal Worker Model is another way to even out the work flow because it inherently reduces waste due to department siloing. In addition, universal workers are able to exercise much more ownership and control over their work areas and, with proper team development and support, reduce the need for extra layers of supervision. These resources can then be re-deployed towards problem solving guides, team trainers, and subject matter experts that bring the latest ideas and knowledge down to the unit or neighborhood level.

LEAN TOOLS

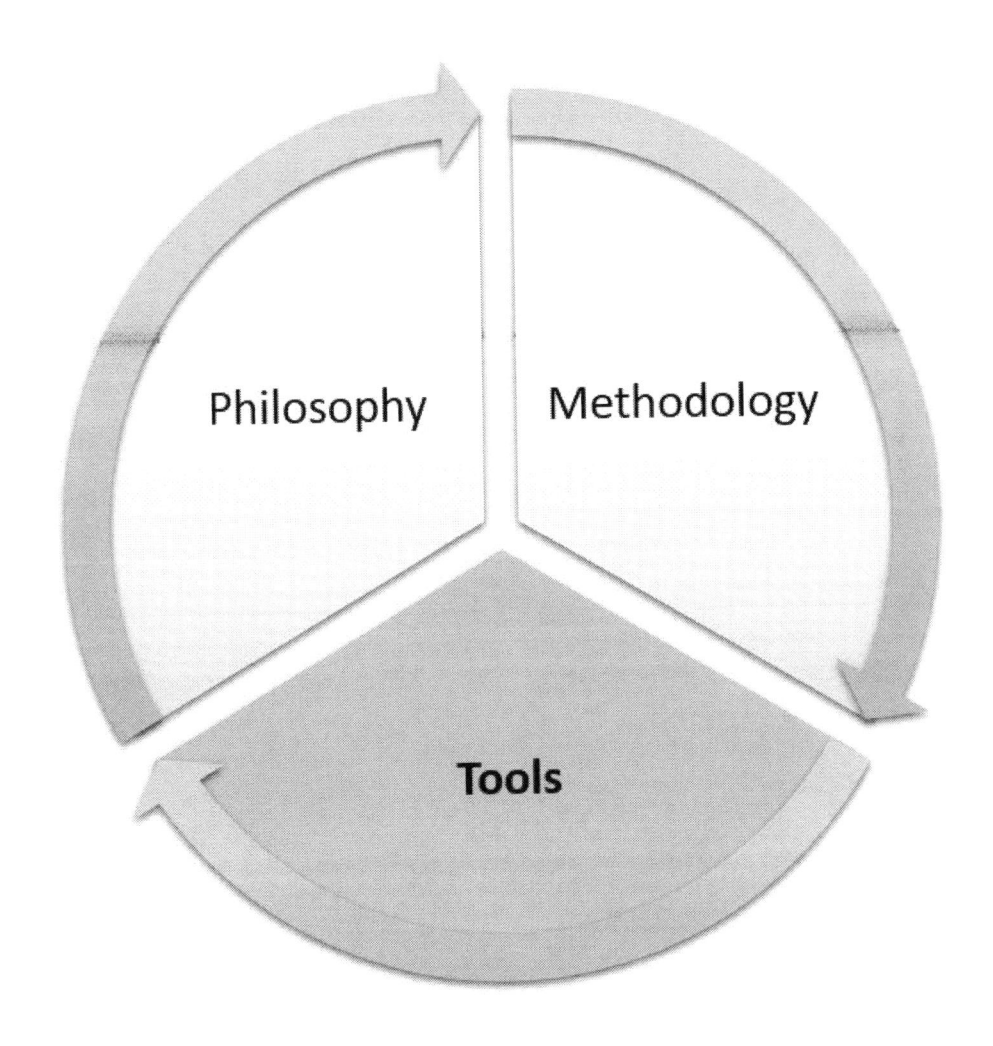

5S

5S is a simple, foundational approach to organizing work areas for efficiency and effectiveness. Because of its simplicity and universal applicability, it's a great first project on the Lean journey. 5S, shortened from the Japanese words *seiri, seiton, seiso, seiketsu,* and *shitsuke*, is frequently translated to Sort, Set, Shine, Standardize, and Sustain. It describes a simple, thoughtful process to organize, clean, and maintain a work area for optimal efficiency.

SORT
Work areas should only contain what is needed. Most work areas, however, are overloaded with items rarely or never used. Sorting items allows you to identify items that aren't used (and dispose of them) or rarely used (and move them). It's tempting to keep items because you "might" need them at some point. Attach a red tag or sticky note to items not used frequently and set them on a designated table. If the item is used in the next month, remove the red tag and keep the item. If not, move or discard the item.

SET
Set (in order) is the organization phase. Everything should have a place, and the places should be determined by the most logical arrangement. Usually this means that objects are organized by type, and rooms are organized by arranging the most frequently used items closest to the person needing them. In a storeroom, this means organizing items in logical groupings and then placing the most frequently accessed groupings nearest the door. While saving a few steps might not seem like a big improvement, its effect can add up.

SHINE
Shine is the cleaning phase. All areas should be clean at all times. Disorganized and dirty areas create waste by obscuring needed items, decreasing workplace safety, requiring additional or repeated cleaning time, or simply by contributing to a disorganized mindset in a team.

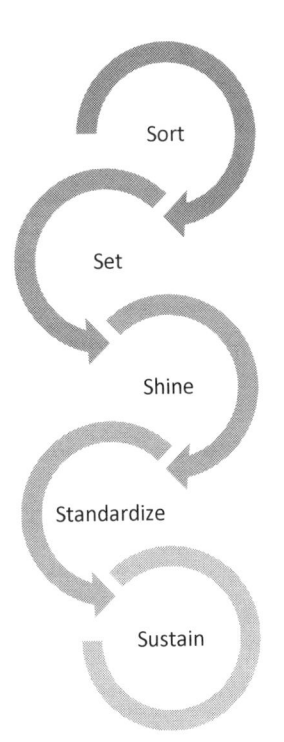

Keeping areas clean can be a challenge when multiple shifts use a single workspace. Let the team decide the best way to share cleaning responsibilities, taking into account usage and the business of each person's day.

STANDARDIZE

Standardization is the labeling and systematizing phases. Items should have clearly marked spaces. Use large, easy-to-read labels and colors to group types or categories. Create keys or legends for large storage areas.

SUSTAIN

The final phase is the most important: keeping an area optimized at all times. Organizing a 5S event is not meant to be an annual "Spring Cleaning." Instead, it should create lasting, sustained organization through design, training, and maintenance. Labels, color-coding, and other systems established in the standardize phase must be kept up. There must be a plan for keeping the area cleaned. Everyone on the team must be trained in not only where to find things, but also how to store things. Finally, there must be routine monitoring and follow-up. This doesn't mean a manager needs to audit a work space or storage area every month. In fact, systems are usually more sustainable when auditing is delegated to team members and rotated. Create a simple checklist and have a different staff member complete it each month.

ORGANIZING A 5S EVENT

Storerooms are the best and easiest place to start. Gather several team member representatives, and clear a block of time to work. Go through the entire storeroom from end to end, applying the steps listed above. A 100-bed nursing home might expect to save $20,000-$35,000 in waste and inventory reduction, in addition to significant staff time savings.

Other useful places to start 5S events are kitchens, housekeeping and laundry areas, medical records storage, treatment/ medication carts, nursing stations, and leisure/ activity spaces.

It's important to note that 5S is not a useful tool unless work teams are involved in organizing and arranging their own areas. Cross-functional and outside perspectives are useful for thinking outside the box and questioning whether an item is really needed, but staff must ultimately take accountability for their own work areas and thus should take the lead during 5S events.

Name: _____

Rate each criteria on a scale from 1 (not at all) to 5 (exemplary)

Category	Criteria	Work Area / Room			
Sort	Is the area free of unnecessary machines/ equipment?				
	Is the area free of unnecessary supplies?				
	Is the area free of broken equipment?				
	Is the area free of outdated supplies?				
	Are notices, memos, signs, etc. current?				
Set	Are all supplies put away?				
	Are supplies arranged first in, first out?				
	Are pathways clearly indicated?				
	Are frequently used supplies easy to reach?				
	Are needed instructions and documents available?				
Shine	Is the work area clean?				
	Is equipment clean?				
	Are walls intact?				
	Are cleaning supplies available and accessible?				
Standardize	Are cleaning assignments scheduled and posted?				
	Is cleaning schedule monitored?				
	Are labels and tags in good condition?				
	Have all new items been categorized properly?				
	Is equipment maintance schedule posted?				
	Is documentation control being followed?				
Sustain	Has all staff been trained on 5S?				
	Are Red Tag Days regularly scheduled and held?				
	Are 5S audits regularly scheduled and completed?				
	Are 5S successes recognized and celebrated?				
	Is management involved in 5S audits and celebrations?				

5S Audit Tool

FIVE WHYS

Asking why will usually get you an answer--- just not always the right one. This seemingly obvious statement led to a practice of asking why five times, or drilling down to uncover root causes of problems, and it is a key part of a successful problem solving process. When we fail to discover root causes, we merely patch over the problem and it likely will seep through another hole. In some cases, failing to find root causes leads to interventions that have absolutely no effect and merely waste staff time and resources.

In long-term care, there is always pressure to resolve issues quickly, usually because there is other pressing work at hand. Unfortunately, this lends itself to a perpetuating cycle of not having time, since problems are rarely far from the horizon. To break the cycle, you must dive deep into problems, find underlying causes, and put in place countermeasures to try and prevent them from reoccurring. Don't let survey agencies or corporate offices shortcut true problem analysis. While a plan of correction may be due to the survey team within a week or two, this doesn't mean that your investigation needs to stop there.

Why ask why five times? There isn't a science to this, nor is it a hard and fast rule; rather, it's a guide to remember to think beyond simple causes and surface explanations. You may only need three or four whys for some problems; other times, you might need more than five. The purpose, always, is to find the root problems to address.

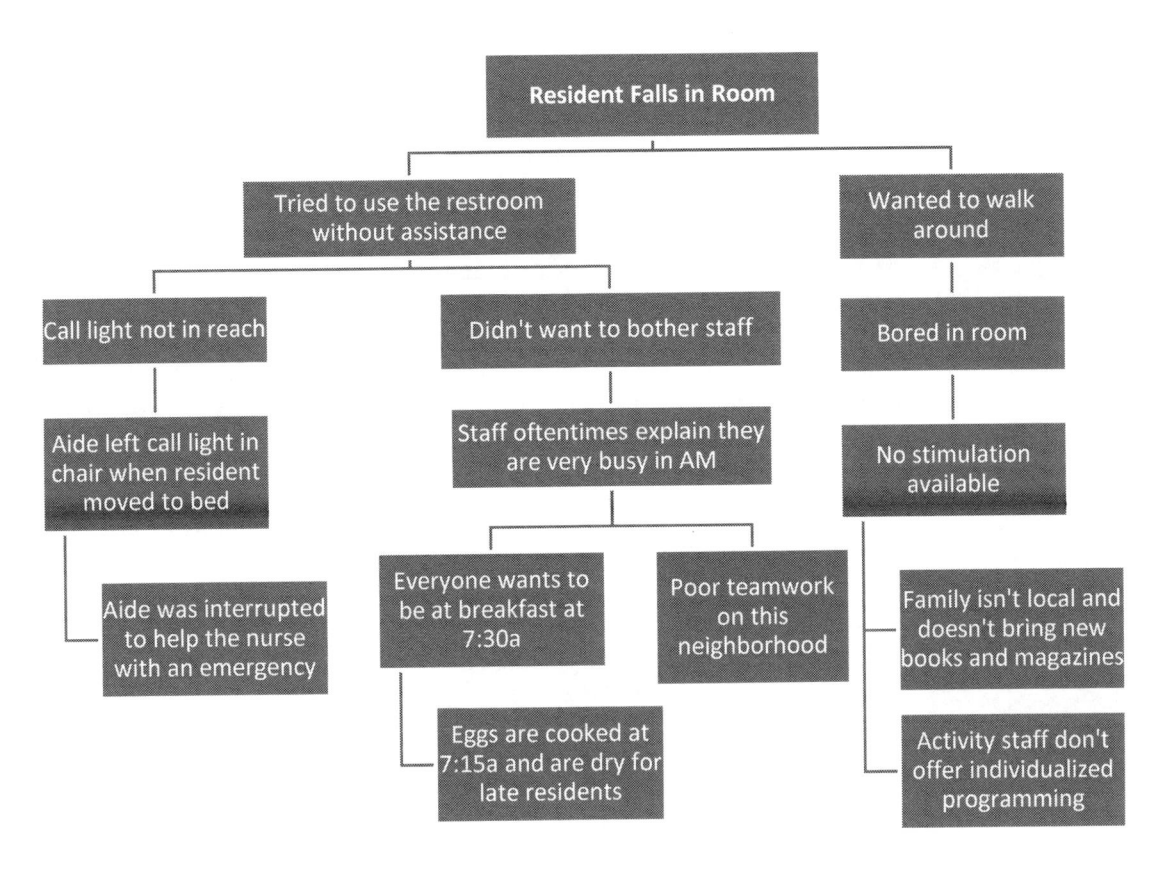

```
                        ┌─────────────────────┐
                        │ Resident Falls in Room │
                        └─────────────────────┘
                          │                │
          ┌───────────────┘                └────────────────┐
┌──────────────────────────┐                    ┌──────────────────┐
│ Tried to use the restroom │                    │  Wanted to walk  │
│   without assistance      │                    │      around      │
└──────────────────────────┘                    └──────────────────┘
          │                                              │
  ┌───────┴────────┐                              ┌──────────────┐
  │                │                              │ Bored in room │
```

- Call light not in reach
- Aide left call light in chair when resident moved to bed
- Aide was interrupted to help the nurse with an emergency
- Didn't want to bother staff
- Staff oftentimes explain they are very busy in AM
- Everyone wants to be at breakfast at 7:30a
- Eggs are cooked at 7:15a and are dry for late residents
- Poor teamwork on this neighborhood
- No stimulation available
- Family isn't local and doesn't bring new books and magazines
- Activity staff don't offer individualized programming

Example of five whys used to determine root cause of a resident fall

So how do you know when you've found the root cause or root causes? Practice, informed thinking, and a little luck. A root cause is the lowest level (most basic) reason why a problem occurs. Root cause analysis, like any skill, is developed over time, and practice, guided by a knowledgeable coach, is the best way to learn. Typically, early practitioners stop too early in the process—another reason to follow the five whys guide—and try to address causes with too many variable underlying causes.

To illustrate this, consider a root cause analysis of a resident fall, diagramed earlier. In investigating why a resident fell in her room, you might discover that her call light was not within reach. If you stop at this point, you might be inclined to discipline the CNA for forgetting this important task. After all, proper placement of the call light is generally considered a standard of practice. By asking why again, though, you learn that the CNA was interrupted to assist a nurse with an emergency, which would probably change the type of intervention to prevent future occurrences.

When investigating root causes thoroughly, you will almost always uncover more than one cause. This is normal because of the complexity in healthcare settings—in fact, an investigation that determines a single root cause for anything but the most mundane of problems should be suspect. In the example above, while the call light not in reach may have been one contributing factor, the investigation also uncovered that the resident was hesitant to use it even when it was within reach because she felt like she was bothering the staff. Again, by digging deep you are better able to prevent issues in the future by developing comprehensive interventions and countermeasures that address the myriad of causes.

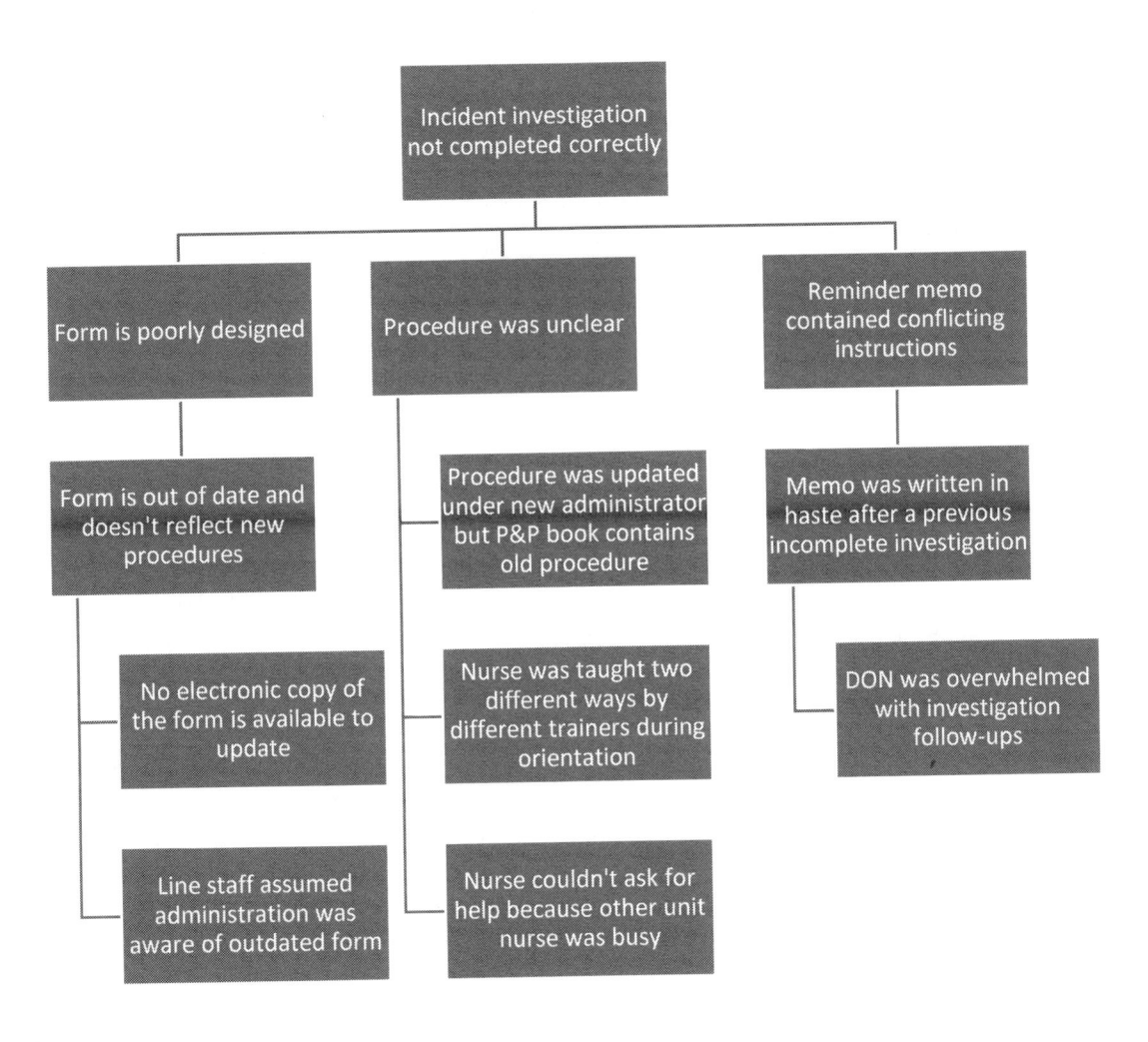

```
                    ┌─────────────────────────┐
                    │ Incident investigation  │
                    │ not completed correctly │
                    └─────────────────────────┘
                                 │
        ┌────────────────────────┼────────────────────────┐
        │                        │                        │
┌───────────────┐     ┌───────────────────┐    ┌─────────────────────┐
│ Form is poorly│     │ Procedure was     │    │ Reminder memo       │
│ designed      │     │ unclear           │    │ contained conflicting│
└───────────────┘     └───────────────────┘    │ instructions        │
        │                        │              └─────────────────────┘
        │                        │                        │
┌───────────────┐     ┌────────────────────┐   ┌─────────────────────┐
│ Form is out of│     │ Procedure was      │   │ Memo was written in │
│ date and      │     │ updated under new  │   │ haste after a       │
│ doesn't reflect│    │ administrator but  │   │ previous incomplete │
│ new procedures│     │ P&P book contains  │   │ investigation       │
└───────────────┘     │ old procedure      │   └─────────────────────┘
        │             └────────────────────┘              │
        │                        │                        │
┌───────────────┐     ┌────────────────────┐   ┌─────────────────────┐
│ No electronic │     │ Nurse was taught   │   │ DON was overwhelmed │
│ copy of the   │     │ two different ways │   │ with investigation  │
│ form is       │     │ by different       │   │ follow-ups          │
│ available to  │     │ trainers during    │   └─────────────────────┘
│ update        │     │ orientation        │
└───────────────┘     └────────────────────┘
        │                        │
┌───────────────┐     ┌────────────────────┐
│ Line staff    │     │ Nurse couldn't ask │
│ assumed       │     │ for help because   │
│ administration│     │ other unit nurse   │
│ was aware of  │     │ was busy           │
│ outdated form │     └────────────────────┘
└───────────────┘
```

Five Whys exercise showing multiple cause chains

FISHBONE DIAGRAM (ISHIKAWA DIAGRAM)

The fishbone diagram is a great way to organize the 5 Whys when dealing with the complex problems present in most organizations. Developed by Kauro Ishikawa, the fishbone organizes causes along separate spokes stemming from the problem. The traditional six "main lines" to consider are:

- People – Anyone involved in the process
- Equipment – All equipment and tools used in the process
- Processes – The process itself, including applicable regulations
- Environment – The physical location, layout, time where the process exists
- Materials – Items used during the process
- Management – The management and oversight system

A fishbone diagram helps to visualize multiple causes of a problem. It also helps to sort causes into similar groupings, and can stimulate deeper thinking about all the factors that might be leading to an observed problem.

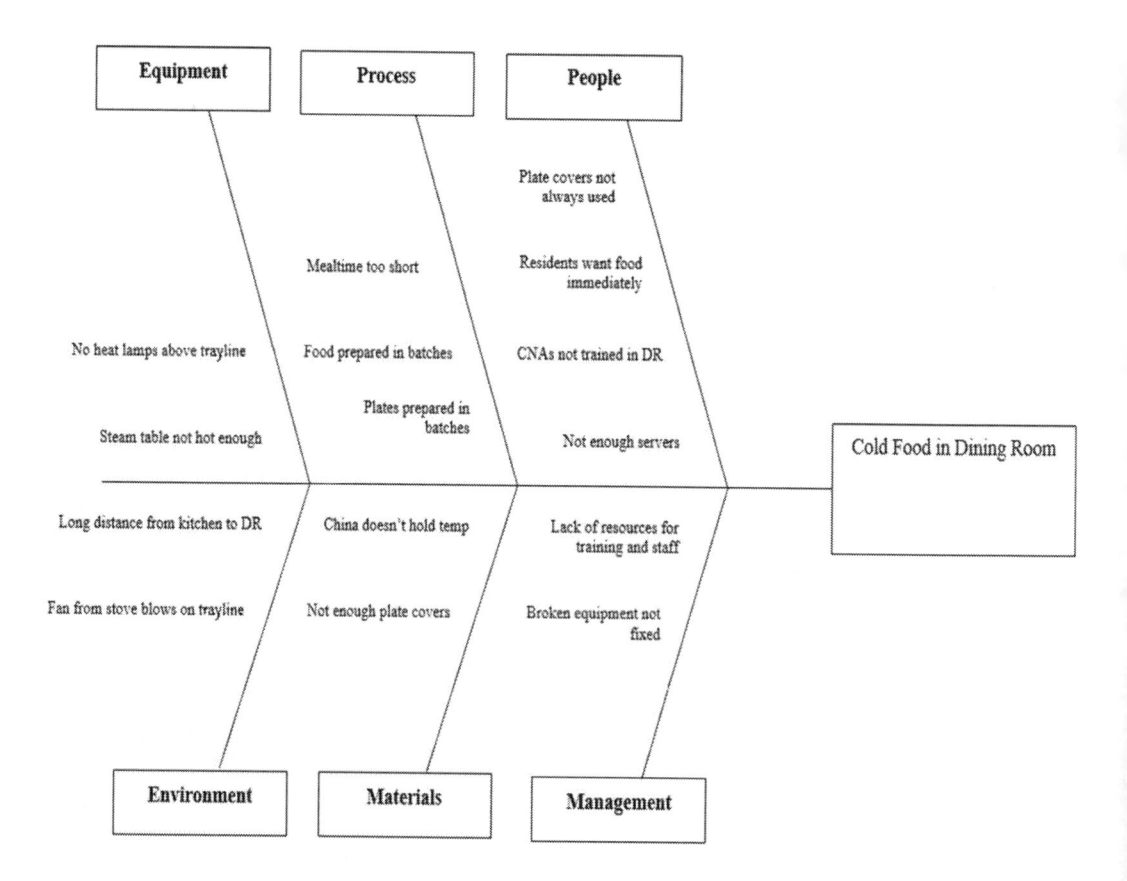

Problem: Cold Food in Dining Room

Equipment
- No heat lamps above trayline
- Steam table not hot enough

Process
- Mealtime too short
- Food prepared in batches
- Plates prepared in batches

People
- Plate covers not always used
- Residents want food immediately
- CNAs not trained in DR
- Not enough servers

Environment
- Long distance from kitchen to DR
- Fan from stove blows on trayline

Materials
- China doesn't hold temp
- Not enough plate covers

Management
- Lack of resources for training and staff
- Broken equipment not fixed

RUN CHART

Run charts display data in a time sequence. They are quite common in healthcare organizations, and are typically used to measure occurrences of events and adverse outcomes, and then determine trends or impact of an intervention. The X axis can be either a count, a percentage, or a rate. Examples might be the number of medication errors, the percentage of completed audits in a neighborhood, or the number of falls per 100 resident days.

Interpreting a run chart is quite straightforward. If you are tracking falls, and the chart is shifting down, this indicates your interventions are possibly having an effect. If there is not a change in the charts, the intervention isn't likely having an effect. You can also use run charts to compare different units or neighborhoods, though it's important to ensure the scale is the same. (The easiest way to do so is to use a rate or percentage to compare, rather than a count, unless the neighborhoods each have the same number of residents.)

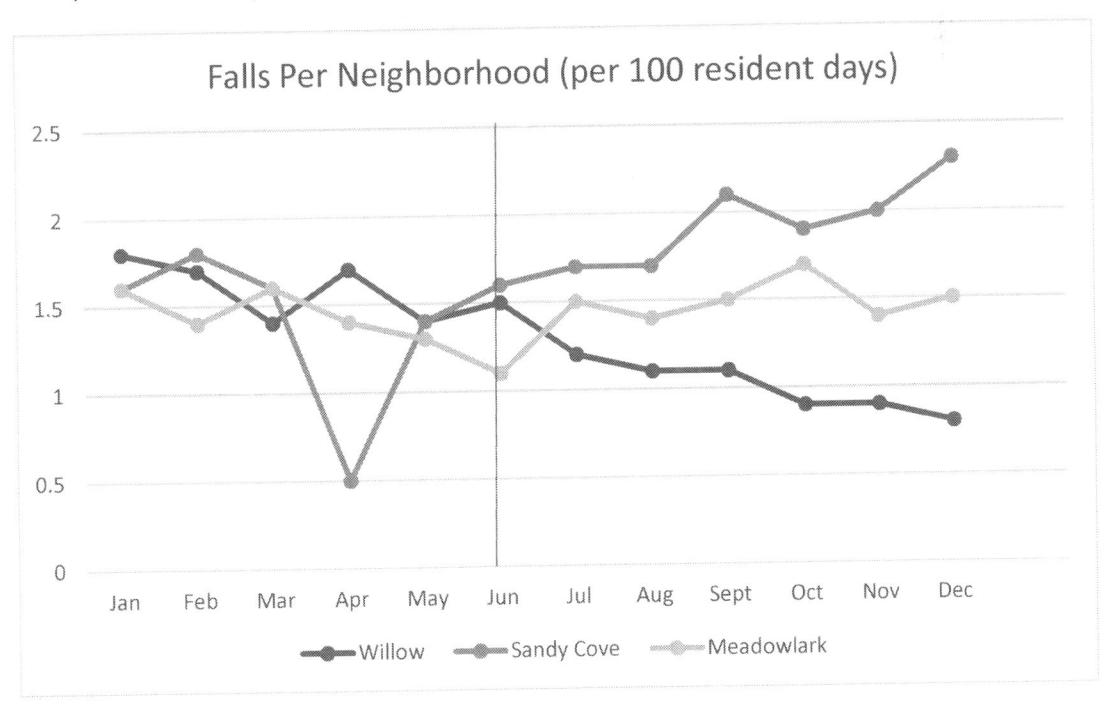

Falls Per Neighborhood (per 100 resident days)

In the chart above, an intervention was implemented in June. Willow shows a solid downward trend, while Sandy Cove shows an upward trend. Meadowlark remains unchanged. Note the sharp drop of falls in Sandy Cove during April. This is called an outlier, which indicates either a problem with the data or a statistical anomaly. In statistical terms, outliers are usually less important than trends, though it's always good to make sure there isn't a problem with the process or data.

CHECK SHEET

A check sheet is a structured form for collecting data in real time. The header contains key information about who is completing the sheet, what was collected, when and where the data was collected, and, oftentimes, why the data is being collected. Check sheets are useful for collecting data to confirm a problem or to examine later during a root cause analysis. By collecting actual data about occurrences, you can better sort out perceived problems or causes from actual ones.

Observer: *Sally Sparkles*, Day
Susie Sprinkles, Evening
Sonny Shining, Night

Date: 7/5/14

Medication Pass Interruption Tally Sheet

Project: Reducing medication errors

Return Form to Laura in Staffing.

Interruption:	Day Shift	Evening Shift	Night Shift
Resident Assistance	IIII	𝐻𝐻𝐻 III	III
CNA Question	IIII	III	I
Nurse Question	𝐻𝐻𝐻 III	IIII	II
Other Question	𝐻𝐻𝐻 II	III	
Answer Phone	IIII	𝐻𝐻𝐻 II	
Med Missing From Cart	IIII	III	III
E-MAR Error	II	III	𝐻𝐻𝐻

PARETO CHART

Not all problems are equally damaging to a community, and not all causes equally lead to a problem. Therefore, it is important to select a few problems or causes (or just one) to tackle at a time. Management Consultant Joseph Juran described the Pareto Principle, or 80/20 rule, based on the work of Vilfredo Pareto, a 19th century Italian economist. He showed that 80% of problems generally come from about 20% of the causes; therefore, it is much more efficient to focus your attention on solving those vital few causes, rather than the other, less common ones. The Pareto chart organizes data by frequency, and provides an easy-to-see view of causes or problems.

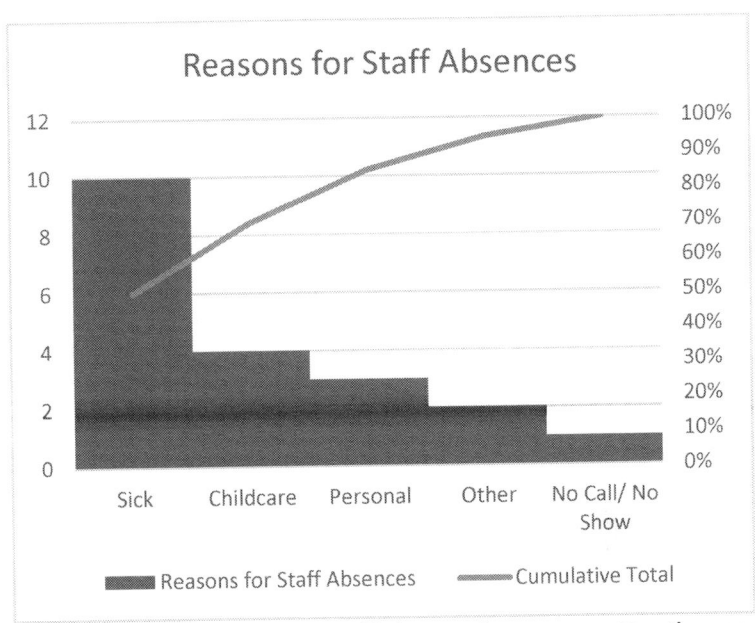

Collect data on a tally sheet, and organize from most frequent to least. The horizontal axis contains the problems or causes, and the vertical axis contains the measurement (count, cost, etc.) This makes it very easy to distinguish the vital few from the useful many.

When analyzing the data, you want to consider the following:

1) Is the right measure being used? Usually we focus on count: how many falls, how many medication errors, etc. However, it might be useful to convert to another scale, such as time spent investigating or cost to the community. Doing so can help uncover hidden waste or better identify the most impactful projects.
2) How many causes account for the majority of the problem? If only one, this is obviously where the team should focus improvement efforts. If there are two or three, you must decide whether to try and address them all, or whether to focus on one at first.
3) Are all causes similar in frequency? If so, you will want to use another type of analysis to determine the focus of improvement activities.

HISTOGRAM

A histogram is a type of chart that shows how data are spread on a measurement scale—basically, a bar graph that helps show how a process or outcome varies. Histograms are easy to interpret, and you can also use them to calculate averages (means), middle points (medians) or standard deviations (how much a process spreads or varies in a statistical way), which can be useful for later interpretation.

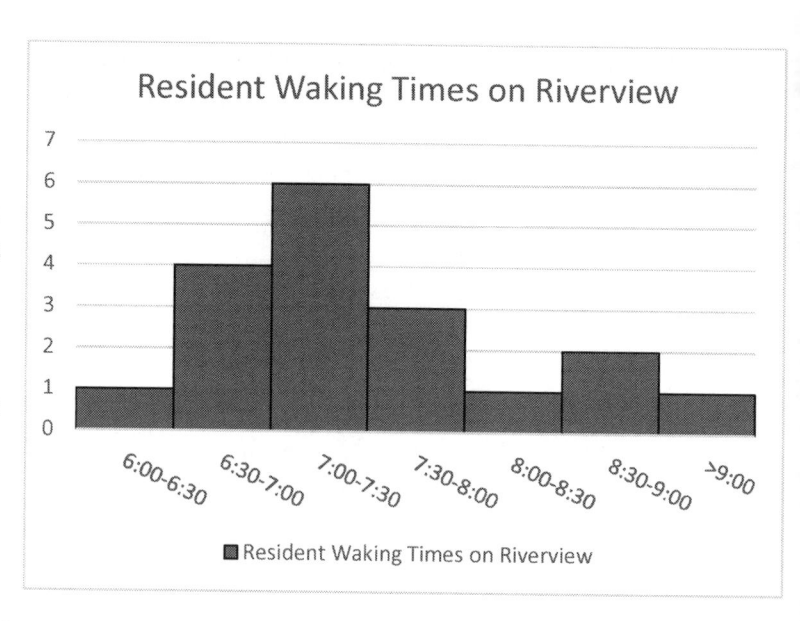

Resident Waking Times on Riverview (histogram with intervals 6:00-6:30, 6:30-7:00, 7:00-7:30, 7:30-8:00, 8:00-8:30, 8:30-9:00, >9:00)

Histograms are easy to construct and one of the most basic tools used in quality management. First, create a check or tally sheet. Next, observe the process and record the data on the sheet. Finally, order the data into equal intervals, create the chart, and interpret the data based on the current understanding of the process.

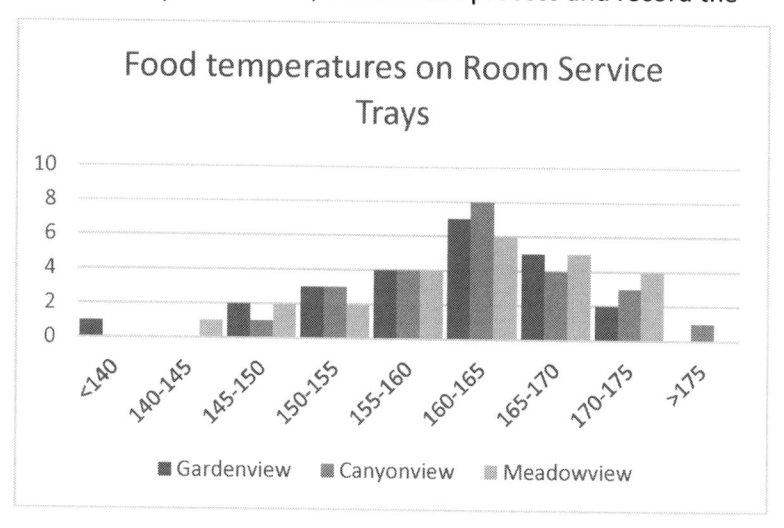

Food temperatures on Room Service Trays (histogram comparing Gardenview, Canyonview, and Meadowview across intervals <140, 140-145, 145-150, 150-155, 155-160, 160-165, 165-170, 170-175, >175)

SCATTER PLOTS

Scatter plots are useful to compare whether two variables are related (correlated, in statistical terms). Scatterplots are useful for analyzing causes determined in a fishbone diagram. You may have heard the phrase before that "correlation is not causation." This means that it's important to apply critical thinking and evidence-based practice when deciding variables to compare.

For instance, you might want to compare the number of medications a resident takes to the number of falls the resident has. One axis contains falls, and the other contains the number of medications. Place a dot where each resident falls on the graph. When the dots are closely ordered around a line, there is some correlation. If there is not a pattern, there is likely not a relationship. Compare the two charts below:

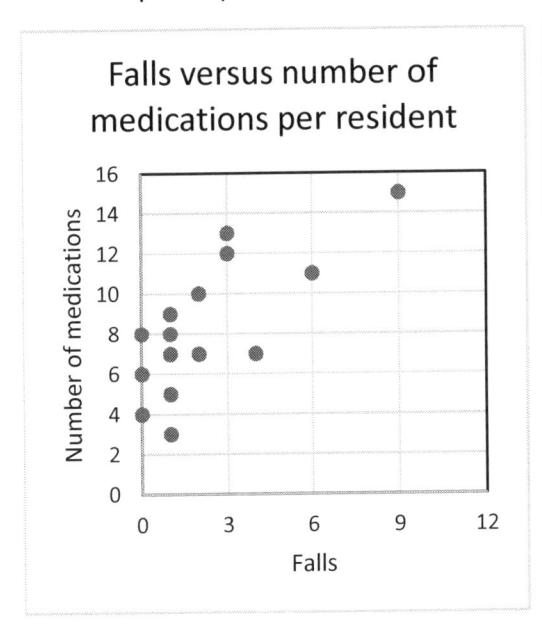

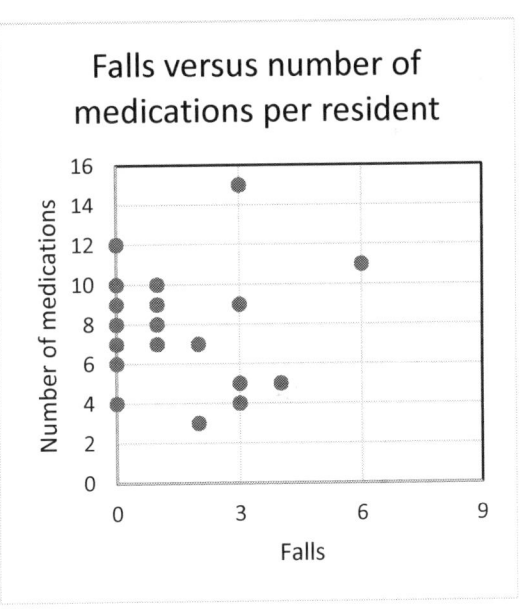

The chart on the left shows a pretty tight grouping along a line. If you are working on fall reduction, a good countermeasure might be to try and reduce the number of medications each resident is taking. On the right side, it shows very little correlation. In this case, you will want to look at other likely causes for falls.

PROCESS MAPS

Understanding process—how work is done—within the organization is crucial to any improvement activity. In fact, it is very difficult to improve any process at all until you understand how it works. Problems sometimes occur because process steps are unknown, even to those expected to do the work. (A CNA who doesn't know about a new infection control procedure.) Other times, processes become mixed up in response to previous challenges. (Staff begin hoarding supplies in inappropriate locations because the supplies are sometimes not available in the storeroom.) Sometimes, variation between individual staff members leads to different processes and outcomes. (Each nurse performing a wound assessment differently.)

Process maps are ways of visualizing a process to better understand the work that is happening. They help to illustrate how information, people and supplies flow, and help describe who does what and when. Several kinds of process maps can be used, depending on the process and goal:

- Value Stream Map: A high-level map of an entire value stream (for example, an admission process from start to finish; a pressure ulcer process from initial assessment to healing; meal service from menu planning to service). Because of their high-level nature, value stream maps can take a lot of time to produce.
- Cross-Functional Process Map: A way to examine a process that is completed by multiple staff and/ or departments. In this map, different people or teams are given a dedicated row, leading these maps to sometimes be called swim lane diagrams.
- Physical Process Map: A process map that follows a process on the floor plan of the building; also called a spaghetti diagram, because staff often walk back and forth. Physical process maps are great for identifying transportation and motion wastes, as well as for redesigning workspaces, storage areas, equipment storage and more.
- Communication Map: A map of the communication lines between people (staff, providers, residents, families, others) during a process. These maps are essential for understanding how information is flowing throughout a process, and can usually identify areas where communication degrades because of the "telephone game" effect (when a message is passed on from person to person and slowly changes).

VALUE STREAM MAP

The value stream map is a comprehensive visual tool to display the flow of information, residents, or services through the series of processes from request to fulfillment. Typically, the value stream mapping process includes a definition of the value stream being analyzed, a map of the current state (done by following the value stream from start to finish), an assessment of the current state (highlighting waste and areas for improvement) and a map of what the future should look like.

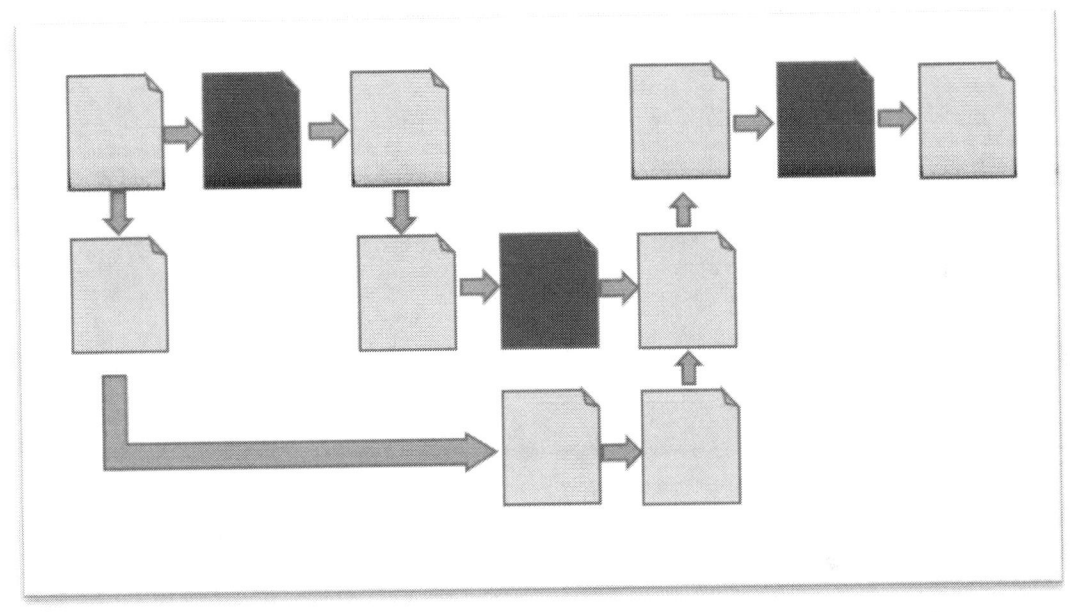

Current state, with problem points shown darker. Note the multiple concurrent processes shown in three levels.

A value stream can be segmented in a couple of different ways. For skilled nursing centers, a crucial value stream would be the rehab guest. The process would start with admission information and end with the discharge summary or conclusion of any post-discharge support. For most aging services organizations, other important value streams will focus on service lines (dining, housekeeping, laundry services, recreation, etc.) or a time period (a very useful value stream is to map a resident day). Sometimes, it may be useful to break up large value streams into smaller portions. Instead of mapping the entire rehab guest experience, you may focus on just the admission or discharge process.

To construct the current state map, start at the beginning of the process. For example, say you want to map the admission value stream. Begin when information about the admission first arrives. Is it an inquiry from a hospital? A tour request from the prospective resident's family? Start in the middle of the page on the left.

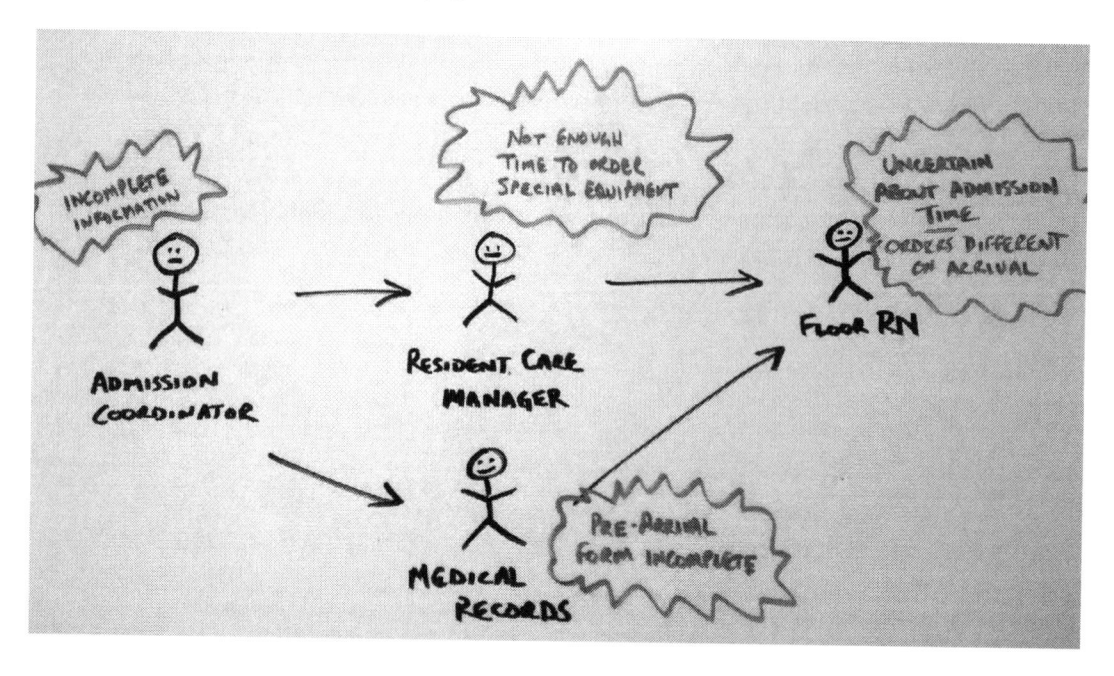

[Figure: Hand-drawn diagram showing stick figures representing process steps. From left to right: Admission Coordinator (with thought cloud "INCOMPLETE INFORMATION"), arrow to Resident Care Manager (with thought cloud "NOT ENOUGH TIME TO ORDER SPECIAL EQUIPMENT"), arrow to Floor RN (with thought cloud "UNCERTAIN ABOUT ADMISSION TIME, ORDERS DIFFERENT ON ARRIVAL"). Below, an arrow from Admission Coordinator goes down to Medical Records (with thought cloud "PRE-ARRIVAL FORM INCOMPLETE"), then arrow up to Floor RN.]

Next, describe each process step, moving from left to right. You probably escort the resident to his or her room, conduct an admission assessment, complete an items inventory, begin the MDS data collection, and so on. If more than one process occurs at once (for instance, medical records being inputted by one department and a care plan being developed by another), draw each additional process directly below. By doing so, you can follow a process linearly as time flows, and see how different parts combine to produce the end result.

You can begin to draw storm clouds in areas where you identify waste or see an opportunity for improvement. (If you are using a computer to map the process, color the problem boxes red.) Say, for instance, there is back and forth dialogue with the hospital discharge planner that delays the arrival. Mark it on the map for future work.

Now, add in information flow. Information flow is recorded on the upper portion of the page, and moves from right to left, showing where the information comes from, who it goes to, and where in the journey it appears.

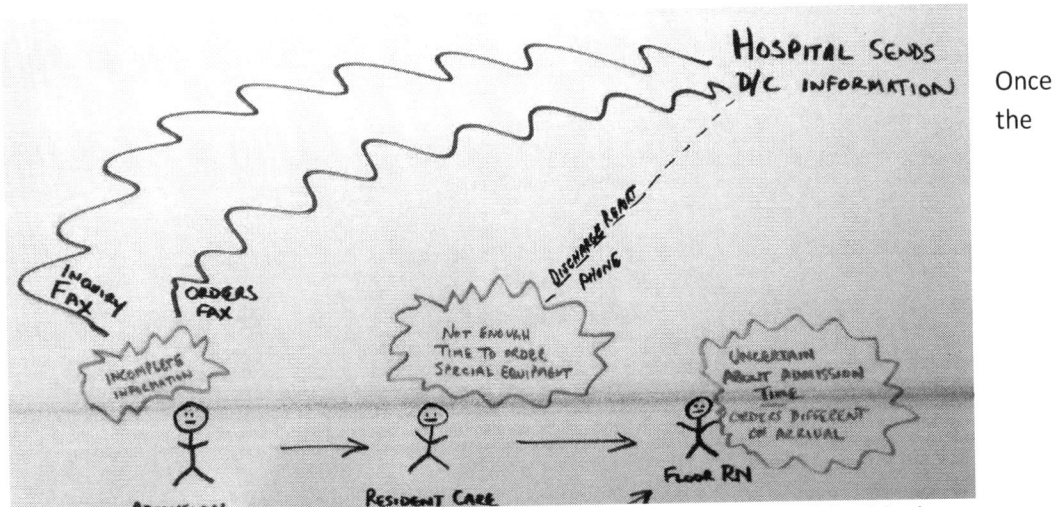

Once the current state map has been constructed and analyzed, create a map of the ideal process. Show how the process could flow if the storm clouds and problem areas were removed. It can be helpful to write each individual process onto a post-it note and arrange them on a wall or board. That way, the improvement team can discuss the order of process steps, and make easy adjustments to improve flow.

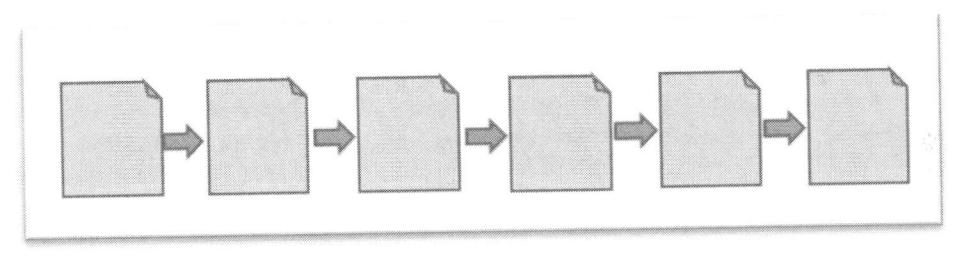

Future state, showing streamlined process

The picture below is a portion of a value stream map developed around a resident day. This map shows residents waiting between tasks (a), process efficiency and effectiveness (b), and value added-time and non-value-added time (c). This version is somewhat technical: C/T refers to cycle time, or the time it takes to perform the work (on average); C/O is the changeover time—the time it takes a CNA to move between residents, including cleanup and walking; FPY is the first pass yield, or percentage of time that the process is done correctly and without errors. While you can dive deep into value stream mapping, most organizations do better to keep it simple at first and not worry too much about standardized markings and formats.

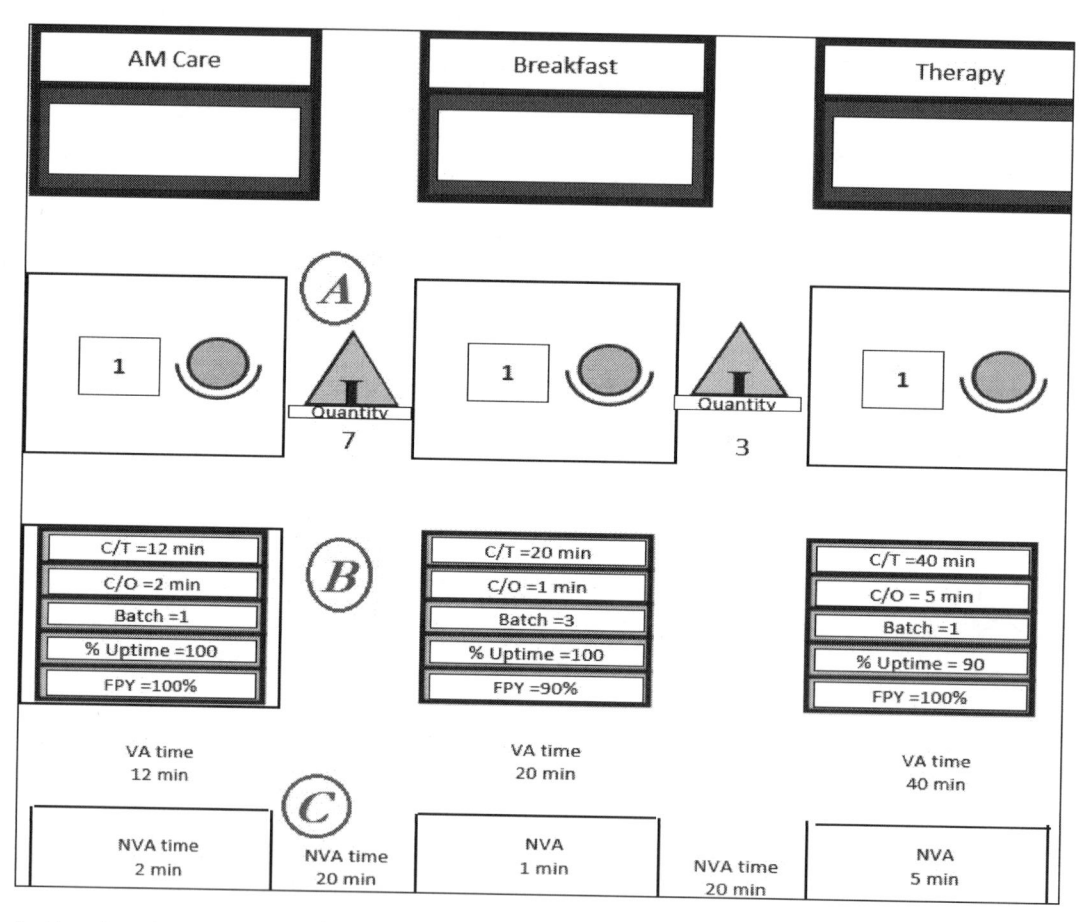

AM Care	Breakfast	Therapy

A

Quantity: 7 (between AM Care and Breakfast)
Quantity: 3 (between Breakfast and Therapy)

B

AM Care	Breakfast	Therapy
C/T =12 min	C/T =20 min	C/T =40 min
C/O =2 min	C/O =1 min	C/O = 5 min
Batch =1	Batch =3	Batch =1
% Uptime =100	% Uptime =100	% Uptime = 90
FPY =100%	FPY =90%	FPY =100%

C

VA time 12 min
VA time 20 min
VA time 40 min

NVA time 2 min
NVA time 20 min
NVA 1 min
NVA time 20 min
NVA 5 min

Portion of a value stream map of a resident day created in SigmaXL

CROSS-FUNCTIONAL PROCESS MAP

A cross-functional process map is a way to organize a process into "swim lanes" that represent different people involved in the process. This type of map is useful to examine cases where a process flows back and forth between people (perhaps indicative of waste), as well as to look at how much time between steps a particular person might spend waiting (useful when trying to level out process flow).

To create the cross-functional process map, make a series of horizontal lines on the chart equal to the number of people (for smaller processes) or workgroups (for larger or more complex processes) involved.

Next, record individual process steps as they occur by moving right when the same person is involved, or up or down if the step is completed by another person. If a large group is mapping the process, consider using sticky notes for each process step. That way, you can easily move, rearrange or add steps if someone realizes that something has been forgotten. Finally, if a process step is a decision, draw a diamond (or rotate a sticky note 45 degrees).

To evaluate the map, consider the following:

- Examine cases where the process flows back and forth between people, and identify ways to reduce the number of bounces. Also, discuss areas where a person or group contributes very little to the process, and see if there are more efficient ways for the process to be completed, perhaps by moving the process step to another person or group. This is a good way to think outside of silos.

- Look at decision points for indicators that someone is checking quality or merely providing oversight. These are good opportunities to build quality into the process and eliminate the check requirement.

- In cases where there is significant wait time between the steps that a person or workgroup is involved in, make sure that their other workload is designed to accommodate this flow. For instance, sometimes maintenance staff set up and break down rooms for events. If there isn't work available during the time of the event, this might represent the waste of waiting.

81

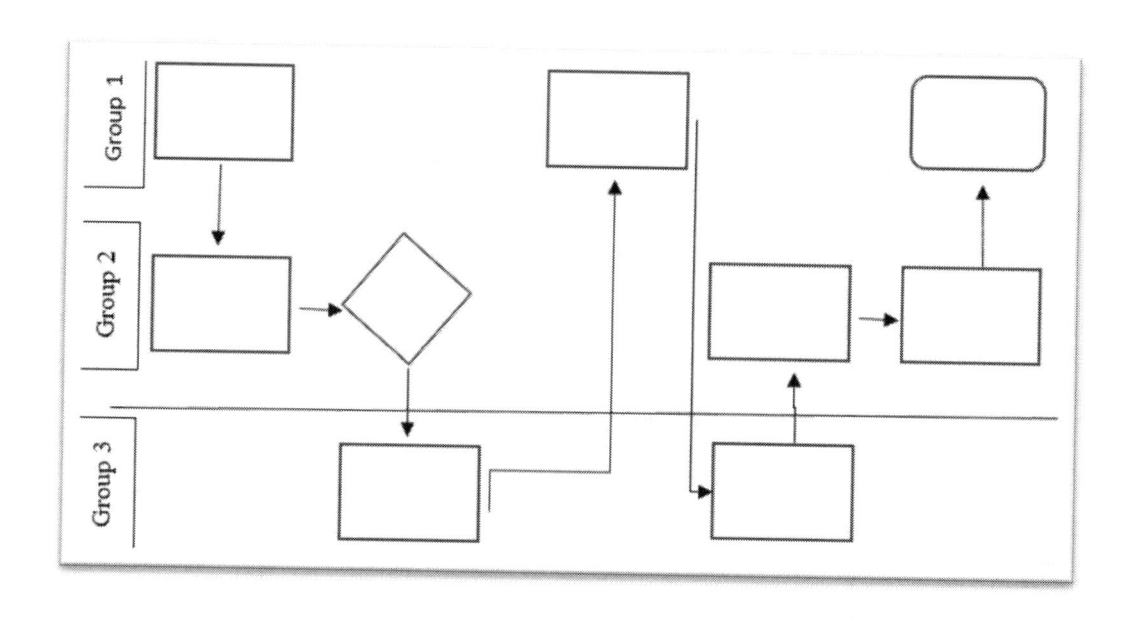

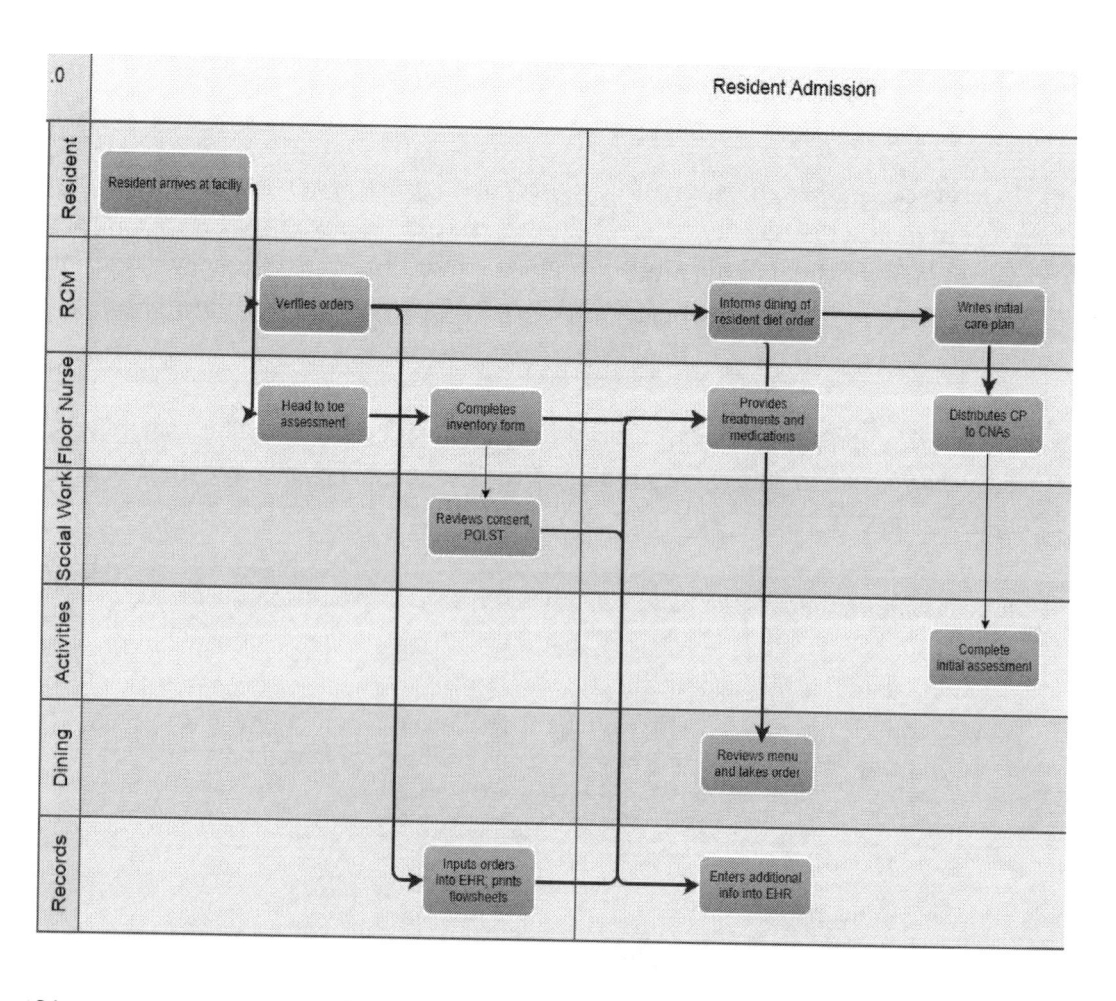

PHYSICAL PROCESS MAP

A physical process map shows how people and things in a process flow through the physical space. Because it generally uncovers a lot of waste around organization and layout, it's frequently referred to as a spaghetti map. The easiest way to create a map is to start with a copy of the floor plan. (Hint: If you're having trouble locating one, look for a fire escape map, which is usually posted extensively throughout healthcare facilities.)

To create a physical process map:

- Mark the first step of the process on the diagram.
- Draw a line or dashed line from this point to the point of the second step of the process. Mark the spot of the second process.
- Continue doing this until you have mapped all steps of the process.

To evaluate the map:

- See what sections of the workspace are not set up optimally. Look for cases where the process loops back and forth over the same path.
- Brainstorm how to improve the layout of equipment, supplies and people to reduce unnecessary walking or transportation. Since physical process maps are visual, they can be left on the wall in a high-traffic staff area (a meeting room, nurse's station, etc.) so that a variety of staff can examine the process map. Sometimes, the most novel solutions come from someone outside of the process offering "fresh eyes."

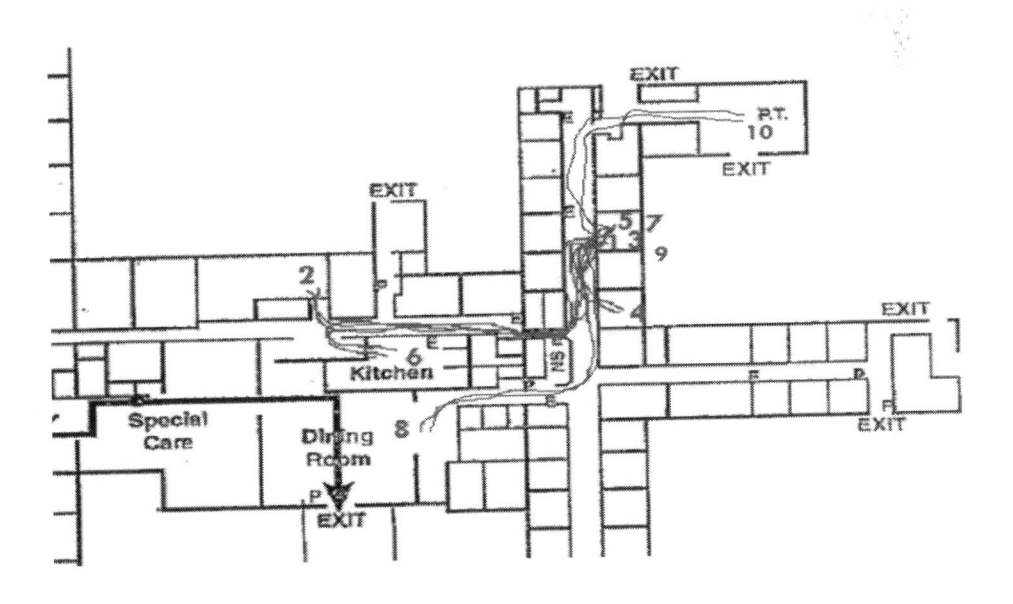

COMMUNICATION MAPS

To illustrate the flow of communication, a modified physical process map can be used.

To create a communication map:

- Instead of using the physical layout, write the names of the parties involved in a process on a large sheet of paper.
- Draw lines between people, with an arrow indicating information flow. When communication between two people occurs more than once, add a hash mark to the line for each instance.

To evaluate the map:

- Look for areas where information is passed back and forth between the same people, or where information might be shared redundantly.
- Consider whether people who might need information in the process are missing from the communication map.

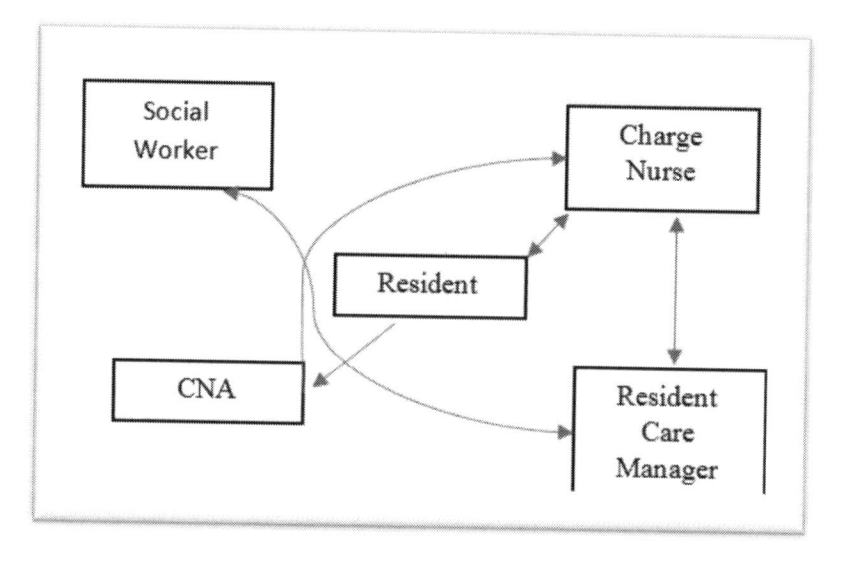

This communication map followed communication of a resident concern that was shared with a CNA. The CNA passed it on to the charge nurse, who talked with the resident and the resident care manager. Finally, the resident care manager and social worker discussed the issue, before communicating back to the charge nurse, who then spoke with the resident. A lot of unnecessary communication and back-and-forth was identified through this map!

RELATIONSHIP MAPS

Understanding relationships in the workplace can be an important component to getting projects accomplished and work done. Perhaps you've experienced an environment where a staff member will listen to some co-workers but not others? Or certain department directors that work really well as a team? Mapping workplace relationships is a strategic way to improve the effectiveness of organizational action.

To create a relationship map:

- Write each person's name and circle it.
- Draw a line from each circle to every other circle, using the thickness of the line to indicate the degree of influence. Each circle should have two lines connected to each other circle (one in each direction).

Optional modifications:

- For a specific project, create a scale of organizational power on one axis and degree of support for the project on the other axis. Place each person on the grid and then connect the lines of influence as above.
- Instead of mapping influence, you can map communication patterns (similar to the communication map above). This is useful in staff meetings to uncover the patterns of staff interactions and can facilitate the creation on effective inter-disciplinary teams.

To evaluate the map:

By understanding which staff are better or more effective at influencing each other, you can build stronger coalitions to enact change.

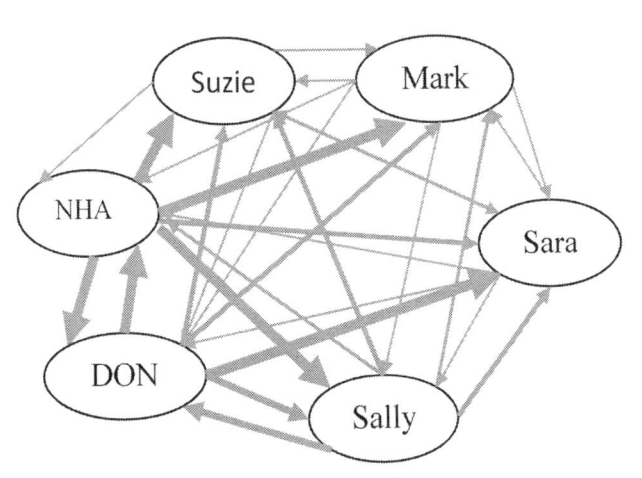

In the relationship map on the left, note how some staff have stronger levels of influence. For instance, while the NHA has strong influence on most of the other staff, the DON has a stronger influence on Sara. Therefore, the DON might be a better choice to approach Sara with a project or new idea. Likewise, Sally appears to have the most influence between herself, Sara, Mark and Suzie, making her a good choice to be a team champion or representative.

GENERATING IDEAS FROM TEAMS

Generating ideas, whether about improvement opportunities or countermeasures to a problem, is one of the most important and under-recognized task of every leader in an organization. It requires attention to the culture and atmosphere at work, support and encouragement to employees at all levels of the organization, and strong systems to sustain creativity and manage follow-up. Alan Robinson and Dean Schroeder note in their book, <u>The Idea-Driven Organization</u>, a steady stream of ideas can lead to competitive advantage, better service and higher quality—three things that aging services providers, now more than ever, must maximize. (Schroeder & Robinson, 2014)

Generating ideas isn't hard and it doesn't have to cost a lot money. In fact, more employees will offer them for free. Why? Humans love to make things easier—it's hardwired into our biology. In a typical workplace, however, rules, bureaucracy, and hierarchies all work to hamper employee engagement and reduce the flow of new ideas. An employee with too many ideas is often ostracized or, worse, accused of being trouble and offered the door. Other employees learn that it's better to be quiet and keep ideas to themselves.

To break this cycle, build a culture where ideas are welcomed. Reward employees for sharing ideas. Create safe spaces when employees' voices aren't overshadowed by louder colleagues or discounted by management. (The nominal group technique can help with this!) Make it easy by ensuring that management spends time with front-line staff in their own work areas. When there, leaders should probe employees, ask questions and encourage contrarian views. Include idea generation and testing in job descriptions and performance evaluations to reinforce its value and importance.

As noted earlier, suggestion boxes are one of the worst methods used for soliciting ideas. Kaizen boards, where ideas and follow-ups are shared openly are much better, especially when working with multiple shifts and departments. Some organizations are starting to use technology, such as idea management software and enterprise social networking tools, to help.

Focus groups and team meetings are great opportunities to solicit ideas from staff or customers (residents, families, other departments, etc.). Techniques for managing ideas are various, but here are a few popular tools:

BRAINSTORMING

Brainstorming is a great way to solicit ideas from a group. A facilitator announces the topic, and participants take turn sharing ideas. The facilitator writes the ideas up on a board.

To be successful, it's important to establish some ground rules:

- All ideas are welcome; no idea is stupid or too crazy
- No criticism of ideas at this stage; only clarifying questions are allowed

Brainstorming is a very simple and easy to use technique for gathering ideas. Its effectiveness can be limited in groups with strong personalities, or new or unfamiliar groups. In these situations, the conversation tends to be dominated by the strongest and most confident voices, while quieter or less assertive voices can remain unheard. In addition, brainstorming tends to lead to "groupthink," where the group narrows ideas for consideration around the themes of the first ones mentioned.

LEARNING CIRCLE

Learning circles are used for both teaching and gathering ideas. Participants gather in a circle. A facilitator announces the topic or question, and passes an object around the group. Each person can either share their thoughts and ideas, or "pass" by handing the object to the next person. No cross-talking or talking out of turn is allowed. After the object has passed around the circle, the facilitator passes it to anyone who passed on the first round and they are given another opportunity to speak (though they can pass again, if they choose).

Learning circles help to reduce power inequalities in groups and equalize voices. However, strong personalities can still dominate the discussion or guide the group thinking in a particular direction.

TRYSTORMING

Related to brainstorming, trystorming involves rapidly coming up with ideas and potential solutions. Instead of spending a lot of time analyzing the ideas or thinking about whether they will work, the group actually tests out a prototype or sample process. This typically involves going out to the area where the work will happen, and creating or performing a mockup. Through visualization of proposed solutions, this helps a team quickly implement plans and is really useful when you have a pretty good idea about the nature of the problem and want to quickly test solutions.

NOMINAL GROUP TECHNIQUE

The nominal group technique is a refinement of the open brainstorming method. A facilitator announces the topic or problem under consideration. Each participant then spends a pre-determined amount of time (usually five or ten minutes) silently writing down ideas. At the conclusion of the silent time, the facilitator goes around the group and each person shares one idea. The facilitator writes the idea on the board and continues until each participant has shared their ideas.

The nominal group technique is also useful for addressing inequity in groups and providing a stronger platform for quieter voices. Its biggest downside is the time required—it can take twice as long as a traditional brainstorming initiative.

Following the discussion of ideas, participants can rank items on a scale or in an order (i.e, either 1-5, or 1, 2, 3...). The idea or solution with the lowest number (i.e. most favored) total ranking is selected as the final selection.

STRUCTURED DISCUSSION

A structured discussion, or focus group, is a useful way to gather information from a group of experts—this could be a group of residents, family members or staff. The facilitator prepares open-ended questions to elicit information, and guides the discussion.

Focus groups can be useful as an independent technique to gain qualitative (descriptive) information from staff or residents. In addition, small focus groups can help inform and guide the creation of surveys and other methods for collecting feedback by bringing your attention to ideas or questions that you might not have considered or by helping to focus previously considered ideas more specifically.

For example, if you were creating a survey for residents or families on your admission experience, a small focus group might give you some ideas about common challenges that they experience. Then, instead of asking a question like, "Did you have any problem during admission?", you could ask, "Did you experience any of the following challenges during admission: (and then list the challenges you heard during the focus group)?" Your survey results will now contain more detailed and specific information that will be easier to act upon.

SURVEYS

Surveys can be a simple and effective way to gather feedback. In crafting surveys, keep questions simple and straightforward. You want to ensure that the responses will provide accurate guidance. Surveys usually have questions that can be answered yes or no, allow the person to indicate their agreement on a scale (called a Likert scale), or are open-ended and allow write-in comments. Yes or no questions provide clear information, but don't always capture the complexity needed with many issues. Scaled questions can help identify overall feelings or patterns of thinking across groups, but don't always provide information on why. Open ended questions provide excellent qualitative feedback (information about what people think), but also tend to have the lowest response rates since they require more effort to complete.

AFFINITY DIAGRAMS

Once a group has many ideas, there undoubtedly will be similarity between some. An affinity diagram helps to organize ideas around common themes. Start by writing each idea on a post-it or notecard, and spread the ideas out on a table. In silence, group members begin moving cards into logical or similar groupings. If it appears that an idea belongs in two (or more) groups, simply write out a second card and place it appropriately.

Once the cards are more or less organized, the group can discuss the groupings, focusing especially on cards that are in multiple places or where there is disagreement between staff. Look for surprising patterns as well.

For each group, try to pick one card that captures the general idea of the group; if none of the cards quite fit, write a separate "heading" card. Finally, arrange the groups into super-groups, if necessary.

MULTI-VOTING

Once you have a large number of ideas, you will need to narrow down choices. Multi-voting is a way to identify top group priorities. Each idea is placed on the board, and participants are given a certain number of votes (usually three or five). Participants mark their vote either by placing a post-it note or a hash mark next to the idea. Tally the votes and select the top ideas to move on to the next stage.

ERROR-PROOFING

One of the key tools in Lean is error-proofing. It's a way of understanding that although humans make mistakes, we can guide behavior and action by indicating a problem (level 1), indicating a problem is likely or about to occur (level 2), and preventing a problem from occurring (level 3). What do these levels look like?

LEVEL 1:

- Fire alarm
- Sterile packaging label
- Alarm on IV pump when empty
- Pressure-sensitive alarms

LEVEL 2:

- Drug allergy warning in EHR
- Using different colors on labels of similar products
- A "confirm" button on EMAR documentation
- "Z-Pak" with day labeling
- Utilizing a checklist for a process or documentation packet
- "Name alert" stickers on the charts of same last names

LEVEL 3:

- Steamer that won't operate with door open
- A mixer that won't start without a guard in place
- Anti-tip wheels on wheelchair
- Pyxis automated medication dispensing system
- Implementing a "Do Not Use" list of problematic medical abbreviations
- Single use safety syringe
- A file cabinet that will only allow one drawer open at a time

Error-proofing doesn't need to be something complicated or expensive. For example, it's common for maintenance staff to be frustrated at having to continually repair wall damage caused by wheelchairs and equipment (especially beds being pushed against the wall). Rather than berate staff, place a protective barrier on high-impact areas. To assist nurses who inadvertently walk away from a computer, add a screensaver lock to prevent protected health information from being visible. If condiments are frequently missing from hallway beverage carts, purchase a holder with a separate space for each item so that missing items are clearly visible.

Error-proofing is NOT idiot-proofing. We don't try to detect or prevent errors because people are stupid or can't do their jobs; rather, error-proofing is a way to ensure that well-trained, committed employees don't make mistakes by accident.

- Make sure that error-proofing isn't being used as a substitute for proper training and orientation to work
- When creating error-proof processes, assume that all errors are preventable
- Consider multiple layers of error-proofing for sentinel-type errors
- Avoid reminding people to pay closer attention (or, worse, putting up a sign telling people to pay closer attention to their work)
- Keep solutions as simple and inexpensive as possible
- Focus on solutions that provide immediate feedback (warning sound, flashing light, etc.) and/ or enable immediate action (process can't continue until the error condition is fixed)

Part of error-proofing is not only responding to mistakes or events, but in examining potential errors, near misses, and close calls. Create a system where near misses are recorded and investigated in tandem with actual errors. The system should include near misses of all kinds, from resident care mistakes to safety hazards to poor documentation. Be sure the system doesn't penalize those who report things—an open and trusting environment, where employees are assured that action is taken based on their observations is key to the program's success. A strong, proactive process of preventing errors will not only improve quality and a resident's experience, it will also save significant time and resources from being diverted to fixing problems after they have occurred.

GETTING STARTED WITH LEAN

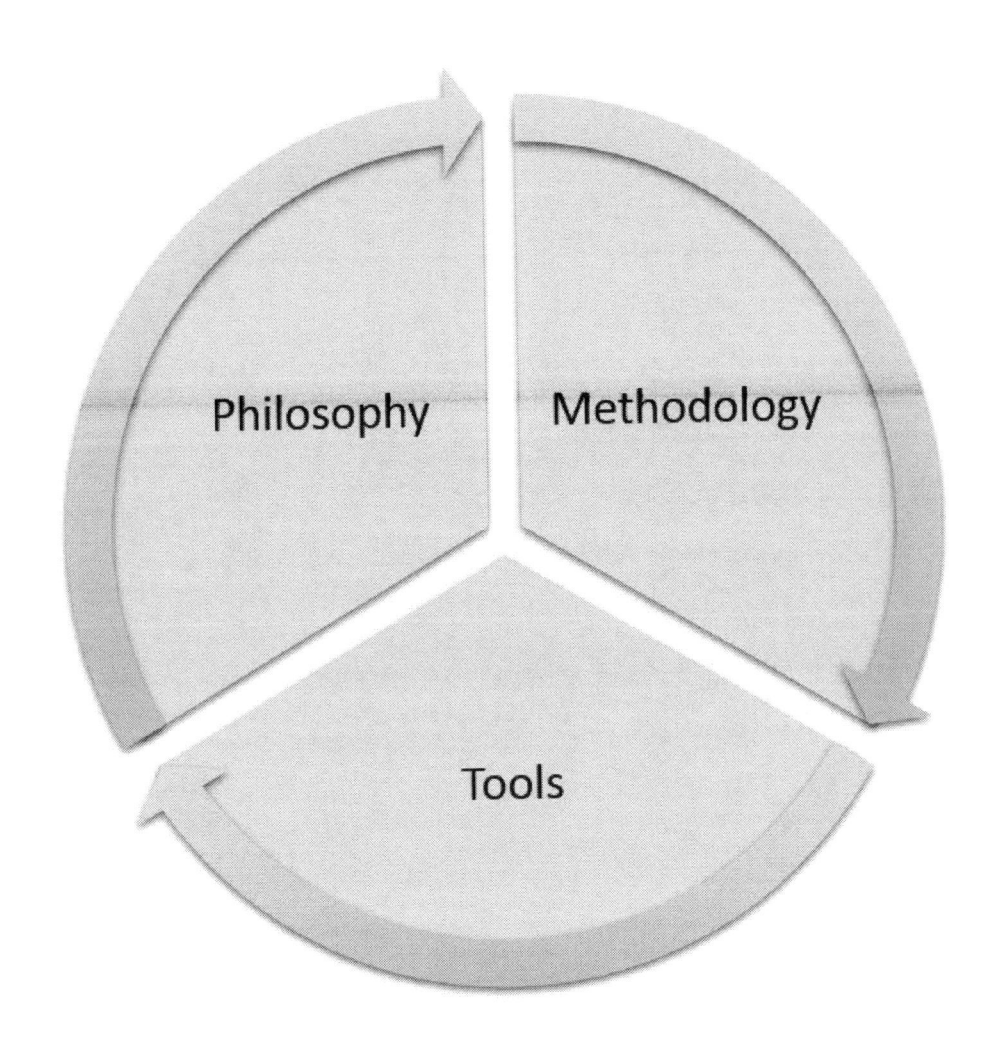

Philosophy

Methodology

Tools

GETTING READY

Hopefully you are excited about the benefits Lean can offer your organization. Before you jump in, it's helpful to step back and do a thoughtful assessment of the organization, workforce, and culture. Otherwise, you'll likely run into a number of bumps during the initial roll-out that can seriously undermine your improvement efforts.

Discovering the level of trust and safety within an organization is a crucial first step. Even if you think you have an open and welcoming culture, it can be useful to conduct some assessments to make sure the rest of the organization (and, in particular, direct care and line staff) feels the same way. A great starting place is to use the Warmth Survey developed by the Eden Alternative. (Eden Alternative) In contrast to traditional satisfaction surveys, the Warmth Survey measures trust, choice, and empowerment, all of which are crucial building blocks for a strong Lean culture.

Psychological safety is another important factor to consider. It's not uncommon for senior leadership to communicate "openness" policies, or encourage anyone to speak up about anything. Leaders may also claim to be transparent, and blame employees themselves when problems are hidden from view. Research has shown, however, that slogans and leadership edicts are not enough to promote a culture of open communication. Instead, power differences between workers and managers need to be considered and addressed, suggestions and commitments need to be followed and tracked, and cultural considerations (not just ethnicity, but also socio-economic backgrounds, prior long-term care experience, and organizational inertia—the tendency for things to stay the same) need to be brought to the forefront. The Agency for Healthcare Research and Quality (AHRQ) has developed several programs around psychological safety and communication in healthcare such as Team STEPPS and CUSP (the Comprehensive Unit-based Safety Program), which are available for free. (Agency for Healthcare Research and Quality, n.d.)

You will also want to review your current quality assurance and quality improvement practices. Look at how the systems identify, track and resolve problems and errors. Look at your current employee training programs, orientation materials, and satisfaction surveys. The audit tool on the following pages can also help position your organization and identify gaps to work on during implementation.

Areas to consider	1	2	3	4	5	Score (1-5)
Leadership Alignment	No leadership alignment for process improvement	Leadership is somewhat aligned with process improvement, but causes substantial review or delay of projects	Leadership aligned with process improvements, but doesn't commit specific resources to projects	Leadership is aligned with specific metrics, and deploys some dedicated resources	Trained and committed resources supporting projects	
Leadership approach towards Lean	Leadership has no understanding of the Lean approach	Leadership has some understanding of the Lean approach, but strong reservations	Leadership has full understanding of Lean approach, but some reservations	Leadership is committed to adopting Lean processes, but not prepared for rapid change	Leadership and organization is prepared for rapid and substantial change	
Prevalent Leadership Style	Authoritarian/ Command and control	Some servant leadership/ adaptive traits, but often resorts to authoritarian practices	Strong servant leadership/ adaptive / collaborative traits, but with unengaged support	Strong servant leadership/ adaptive / collaborative traits with partial engaged support	Strong adaptive traits with consistently strong support	
Leadership Availability	Little to none; unwelcoming/ unpredictable mood swings, closed office door	Some; sometimes unwelcoming or frequent closed office door	Some; welcoming, but frequently unavailable; office door usually open	Good; welcoming and usually available; office door almost always open	Excellent; welcoming and proactively available; office door consistently open	
Leadership Factors						
Employee Engagement	Little to no engagement of employees; frequent inter-staff unresolved conflict	Some engagment, but poorly developed systems; frequent inter-staff conflict	Partial engagement with some systems (forums, learning circles); minor conflicts	Good engagement with active feedback systems and positive team dynamics	Excellent engagement with formal and active systems; rare unresolved conflict	
Employee Involvement	Little to no involvement in improvement work	Some involvement in improvement work (mostly within departments)	Some inter-disciplinary improvement work	Improvement work is structured and driven by inter-disciplinary teams; some formal authority lacking	Leaders and line staff fully involved in improvement; staff empowered to enact changes	
Training/ Education	No training on Lean or quality improvement practices	Few team members have limited or informal training in Lean	Team members are trained in basic concepts like 5S, Lean overview	Team members have good understanding of process improvement methodologies	Process improvement work is integrated in daily flow	
Standardized Work	Policies and procedures are out of date and unused	P&Ps current, but updated by management staff only	P&Ps current and developed with staff input; process for ensuring accuracy	Standard work procedures are current and posted in appropriate areas	Employees have quick access to all standardized work and fully understand process for updating as necessary	
Employee Factors						

Areas to consider	1	2	3	4	5	Score (1-5)
Approach to Errors	Acceptable and/or expected; rely on oversight and auditing; deal with customer complaints	Although errors happen, some initial thought prevails to implement or design error-free systems using Lean	Inspection and control systems only; some data-driven improvement work	Errors are routinely analyzed for system-level problems and causes	Error reporting is non-punitive; focus is on error-proofing and system building	
Data-driven Problem Solving	Insufficient data available for key processes needing improvement; most data is collected for CMS purposes	Organization rarely uses data driven problem solving methods. Data collection processes are not systemic	Organization uses data driven problem solving methods. Data collection is systemic/efficient, but retrospective	Data analysis used to drive some prospective or predictive planning	Virtually all decisions are data-driven; strong data collection systems support predictive action	
Continuous improvement culture	No formalized improvement methods exist outside of QA committee. Staff not concerned with continuous improvement	Improvements reactive – usually come from QA or resident complaints. Some formal employee training in problem solving	Some improvement methodology evident; teams sometimes used to develop solutions. Formal training supported by management	All employees trained on continuous improvement. Methodology evident in most work areas	Methods such as PDCA are known and used by all employees; continuous improvement is a part of evaluations and standards	
Problem Solving Factors						
Finance Support for Lean	Financial oversight is poorly developed or not timely	Financial oversight is timely, but only retrospective; emphasis on cost containment and meeting budget targets	Financial oversight considers long-term implications; cost accounting includes understanding of Lean concepts	Finance office aligned with Lean concepts; some work on budget support for Lean programs	Financial, cost accounting and budgeting processes fully integrate Lean concepts	
Organization of work areas	Messy, no formal workplace organization standards, materials have multiple locations	Some areas well-organized, but no systemic assessment or improvements	Most areas organized, some assessments and walk-thrus present	Training on 5S and related concepts	5S fully implemented and sustained in all work areas	
Other Organizational Factors						

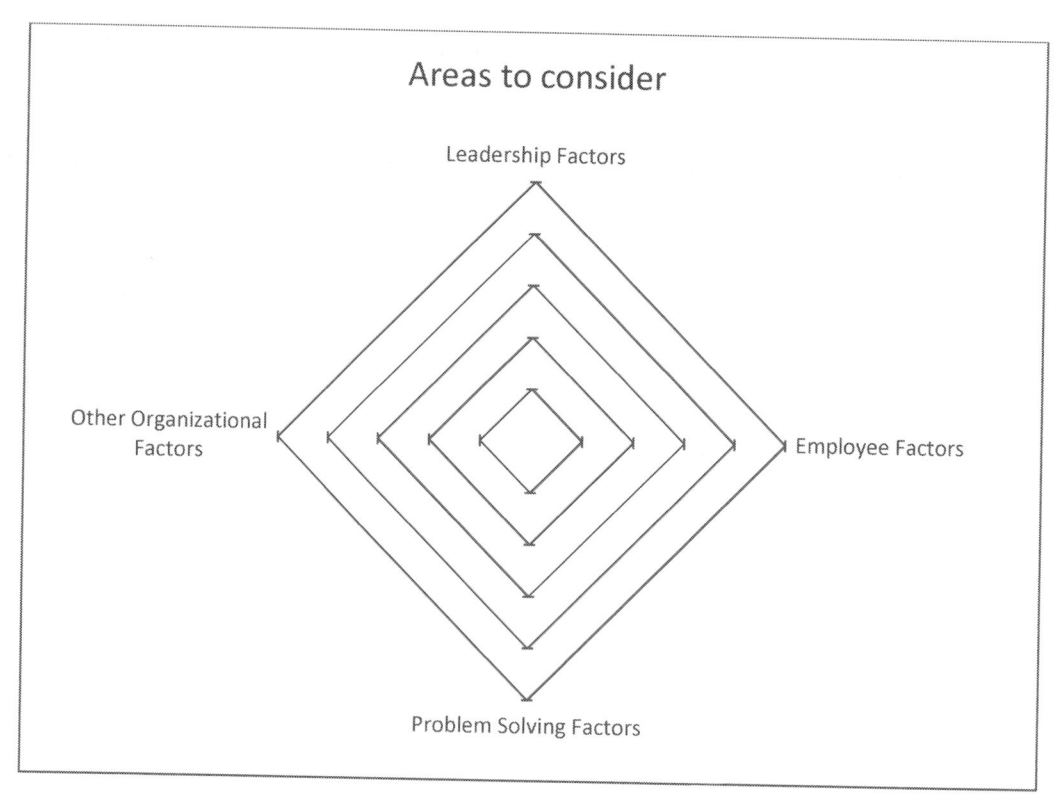

Areas to consider

- Leadership Factors
- Other Organizational Factors
- Employee Factors
- Problem Solving Factors

Instructions: Score each item on the preceding two pages. It is sometimes helpful to have a team score the items, and then average the scores. Next, total the scores for each section. Divide the total score by the number of items in the section. For example, the leadership factors section has four items, so you would divide the total by four. Plot the result on the chart above.

This grid can be useful for positioning the organization and guiding implementation resources. An example is below:

4	5	Score (1-5)
hip is aligned with etrics, and deploys dicated resources	Trained and committed resources supporting projects	2
ip is committed to ean processes, but ed for rapid change	Leadership and organization is prepared for rapid and substantial change	1
ervant leadership/ collaborative traits al engaged support	Strong adaptive traits with consistently strong support	2
coming and usually office door almost ways open	Excellent; welcoming and proactively available; office door consistently open	3
		8
agement with active ystems and positive	Excellent engagement with formal and active systems;	2

Areas to consider

- Leadership Factors
- Other Organizational Factors
- Employee Factors
- Problem Solving Factors

In this example, the organization scored relatively well on problem solving factors and weakest on leadership factors. This can help inform the program development by showing that the organization should focus initial efforts on building the Lean knowledge of leadership staff and changing management behaviors to build a firm foundation for success.

NEW BEGINNINGS

Hopefully Lean sounds like something that can dramatically help your community: improvement, respect, increasing value and reducing waste—there's a lot to like, for sure. If you are like most people in aging services, however, you're probably wondering where you'll find the time. With so many projects going, daily work to complete, and fires to put out right now, there usually isn't even time in the day for regular work, let along another big idea.

In addition, a Lean program is unlikely to be the first large initiative rolled out in your organization, and some staff will probably approach the new program with skepticism. It's okay to acknowledge past program failures, as well as candidly share that you expect bumps in the future as well. Lean is a continuously improving system. Focus on your commitment to the pillars of Lean: constant improvement, respect for people, and long-term vision. Begin to create a culture where mistakes and challenges aren't feared, but rather accepted—and even welcomed!

Encourage team members to bring their concerns to you. Encourage employees to help identify ways that the organization is struggling to embrace Lean and then involve them in improving the approach. The best organizations in the world don't begin that way—they work hard to continuously improve and constantly adapt. Lean provides a strong set of tools, a solid approach to problem solving, and a core philosophy that can transform your community into a world-class organization.

Now it's time to get started!

LEAN AND QAPI

Lean is a perfect program to adopt for compliance with the upcoming CMS mandate for QAPI (Quality Assurance and Process Improvement). By combining a rigorous, resident-centered process improvement philosophy with existing quality assurance program data, providers can not only meet CMS regulations, but also generate true value for residents by focusing on meaningful quality improvement and waste reduction in the pursuit of excellence.

LEAN AND THE FIVE ELEMENTS OF QAPI

ELEMENT 1: DESIGN AND SCOPE

Lean, by design, encompasses an entire organization and becomes engrained in the organization's core leadership and mission. Providers must commit to relentlessly eliminating waste by practicing continuous, systematic improvement. By promoting a culture of improvement and developing people to understand and create more value in their work, a Lean approach also helps ensure "everyone is on board."

ELEMENT 2: GOVERNANCE AND LEADERSHIP

QAPI requires that the governing body and administration commit both in writing and in practice to a culture of quality improvement and excellence. A Lean program starts with acceptance and promotion by the governance structure and is most successful with active administrative support. Lean takes leadership a step further and commits to a method of problem solving that respects people and creates lasting value in pursuit of the organization's mission.

ELEMENT 3: FEEDBACK, DATA SYSTEM, AND MONITORING

Built on the principle of continuous improvement, Lean provides a rich framework to monitor quality, measure improvements, and maintain gains. By focusing on data, Lean is primed for compliance with QAPI. And by creating systems of quality and cultures of active participation and respect, Lean can help organizations move beyond traditional nursing metrics to seize opportunities for value creation in dining, marketing, and ancillary services.

ELEMENT 4: PERFORMANCE IMPROVEMENT PROJECTS

By using A3s or other documentation of PDSA cycles, improvement activities will already be organized into measured, documented projects in compliance with CMS standards. But project-based improvement is only the beginning: Lean creates an engaged, responsive workforce that actively seeks out opportunities for continuous improvement. No more waiting month-to-month for a QA committee to test improvements and evaluate residents; Lean empowers each employee to contribute to a stronger, more productive organization.

ELEMENT 5: SYSTEMIC ANALYSIS AND SYSTEMIC ACTION

Lean culture, through documented quality improvement, ensures an organization moves forward. As hospitals and health systems look more and more to partner with organizations that can prove their value, a Lean base provides hard data on organizational excellence. Further, the program allows organizations to quickly attack any problem area with a focused, universal improvement discipline, increasing teamwork across functional silos and generating a stronger sense of togetherness across the organization.

MAKING A LEAN PROGRAM QAPI COMPLIANT

In order to fully comply with QAPI guidance, a Lean program must be formally chartered from the governing body (either the Board of Directors or the corporate parent). The charter should include a statement of purpose and assign accountability to a senior leader. The program's scope should at least include an entire community—though the benefits of lean are magnified when deployed throughout an entire organization.

Job descriptions must be updated to include improvement work expectations for each job role. Facility policies should describe how Lean initiatives align with regulatory requirements like resident care, quality of life and community operations. A3s and other documentation of improvement projects should be maintained for survey auditing purposes.

For more information, tools, and templates, visit the official CMS QAPI website: http://www.cms.gov/Medicare/Provider-Enrollment-and-Certification/QAPI/nhqapi.html

WHERE TO BEGIN

After you have warmed the soil by assessing your current culture and alignment with Lean, it's time to pick a pilot area to begin the training. Select a team—either a nursing neighborhood, a floor, or a department—that is highly engaged and energized about making things better.

It can be tempting to educate staff first on Lean tools and jump into improvement projects. A more sustainable approach is to spend time educating staff on Lean philosophy and methodology first, and then move into tools. This is also a good time to start rolling out updates to personnel policies that may have been punitive or disengaging, such as incident investigations, work standards, attendance, et cetera. It's important to not only talk the talk, but also walk the walk.

Once you have provided some initial training, select a simple improvement project to tackle. Use an A3 report to work through the problem-solving steps, educate staff as needed on improvement tools and techniques, and provide support and mentoring as the team identifies the root cause(s) and implements counter-measures.

It's normal for the team to struggle and attempt to revert to old ways by seeking answers from the leadership team. When this occurs, provide additional training, review their process steps, and help them return to the improvement process. Remember: the team learns very little if you provide answers. The role of a Lean leader is to teach the process, empower the people, and remove barriers to the team as needed.

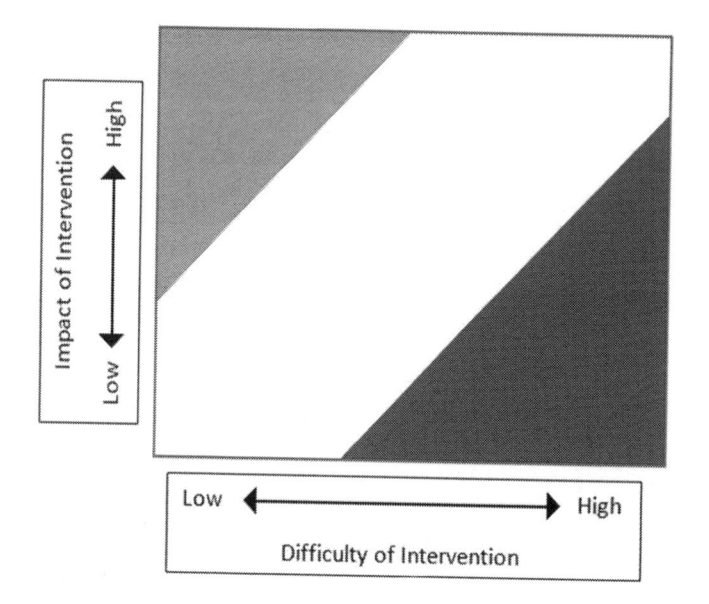

IMPACT VS DIFFICULTY

With so many different challenges to tackle, it can be difficult to know where to begin. And once you begin a project, sometimes it's tough to know which interventions to try first. One way to sort out either issue is to construct an impact/difficulty matrix. With each project or intervention, consider how much of an impact it will have. For instance, a project to improve food temperatures might have a much higher impact than a project to improve the supply ordering system. Next, consider how difficult the project or intervention is to implement. Updating a form is relatively easy, but remodeling a dining room would be quite difficult. When thinking about the difficulty, carefully consider factors such as resource availability, staff attitudes towards the change, and external forces of support or opposition.

By plotting items on the matrix, you can make an informed decision about where to devote your resources. In the matrix on the previous page, the top left shaded area is the high impact, low difficulty portion. Items in this area are called low hanging fruit, and should generally be picked first. The bottom right section is low impact, high difficulty items. Items in this area are generally not worth the investment, unless other options have proven unsuccessful.

In another version of the chart, ideal for project sorting, a series of boxes indicate 1st, 2nd, and lower priority initiatives. The top, left corner are projects to tackle first, and the middle box lists projects to begin next. The bottom right area is great for ideas to keep on the back burner, when there is spare time to dream, or to keep an eye on if the difficulty or impact changes. New technology, as one example, frequently allows once impossible changes to be made, so it's a good idea to never completely rule an idea out.

Improvement projects should also fall in line with organizational goals and overall strategy. This is why alignment in all areas of the organization is crucial to organizational efficiency. If the organization is struggling with a low census, projects that impact satisfaction and marketability will be more crucial than projects that target less critical service areas. After a poor survey, projects almost certainly will focus on quality issues that need attention. One of the advantages of Lean long-term is that problem solving becomes a part of everyone's daily routine. This allows a Lean organization to tackle much more improvement work at one time than an organization where only a few select individuals are responsible for change activities.

102

PROJECT COMMUNICATION (RACI MATRIX)

Teams need to communicate with a variety of stakeholders who will not be involved directly on the team. A responsibility assignment, or RACI matrix, can help define who needs to know what. It's a good way to map out various stakeholders, helping to ensure everyone is involved as appropriate. RACI stands for Responsible, Accountable, Consulted, and Informed. (Smith & Erwin)

- Responsible ("The Doer"): These people are assigned work tasks to complete. Oftentimes, responsible parties are part of the project team, since they will be completing the work.
- Accountable ("The Buck Stops Here"): This person is ultimately answerable for the project, and assigns tasks to those responsible. This is usually the project sponsor or the Administrator, Director of Health Services/ Nursing or other key position.
- Consulted ("In the Loop"): These people are generally department managers or other knowledgeable staff members who will weigh in before final decisions are made.
- Informed ("Good to Know"): Generally, this category is for anyone who will be affected by the project or the outcome. It's important to communicate to this group the status of the project and any resulting changes, but otherwise their input isn't required.

Task ⌄ Role >	Administrator	DNS	Mary-RN	Sandy-CNA	Suzie-Staffing	CNA Group	Nurse Group	Exec Office
Organize staff learning circles	A		R	R	R			
Revise Fall P&P	A	R	C	C		I	C	
Distribute letter to families	A/R	I	I				I	I
Discuss at resident council	A	R		R				I
Remove alarms from Meadowview	C	A/R	R	R	I	I	I	I
Review fall data	C	A/R	R	R				I

The matrix helps to ensure activities are completed, stakeholders are involved and notified as needed, and projects don't stall due to unclear roles and responsibilities.

FORCE FIELD ANALYSIS

Implementing new programs or ideas can be very challenging. One way to strategize towards a goal is to examine the forces that favor the change (the driving forces) and the forces that are opposed to it (the restraining forces).

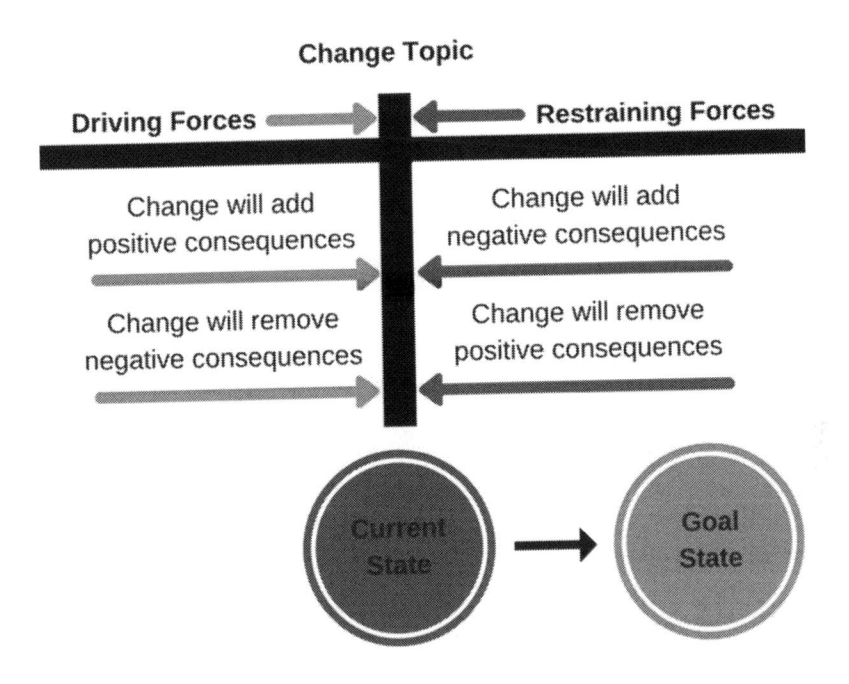

Change Topic

Driving Forces → ← Restraining Forces

- Change will add positive consequences
- Change will add negative consequences
- Change will remove negative consequences
- Change will remove positive consequences

Current State → Goal State

In a stable system, the driving forces and restraining forces are in balance. In order to successfully make a change to the system, the driving forces must be increased, the restraining forces must be decreased or both must occur.

To conduct this exercise, draw a large T and write the proposed idea or change on top. On the left side of the line, write out the driving forces behind the change. Examples might be a market need for a new program or a corporate directive to implement a program. Perhaps residents desire a change in the meal offering. On the right side, write out the restraining forces. Examples could be a limited budget, a staff member who is very committed to an existing system he designed himself, or an outdated kitchen.

By examining the driving and restraining forces in detail, it becomes easier to find levers—particular people or aspects in the system—that can be moved to push forward the overall change. The force field analysis tool is also useful for identifying major barriers to a change or highlighting important reasons that change is necessary that might better inform strategic planning or help determine the right time to make the change.

GANTT CHART

A useful way to plan a project with multiple, overlapping timeframes is to use a special kind of bar chart called a Gantt chart. These charts show the beginning and end of a project task, and organize them horizontally in terms of sequence. This helps to organize projects that have multiple, overlapping pieces, some of which are required before future tasks can be completed.

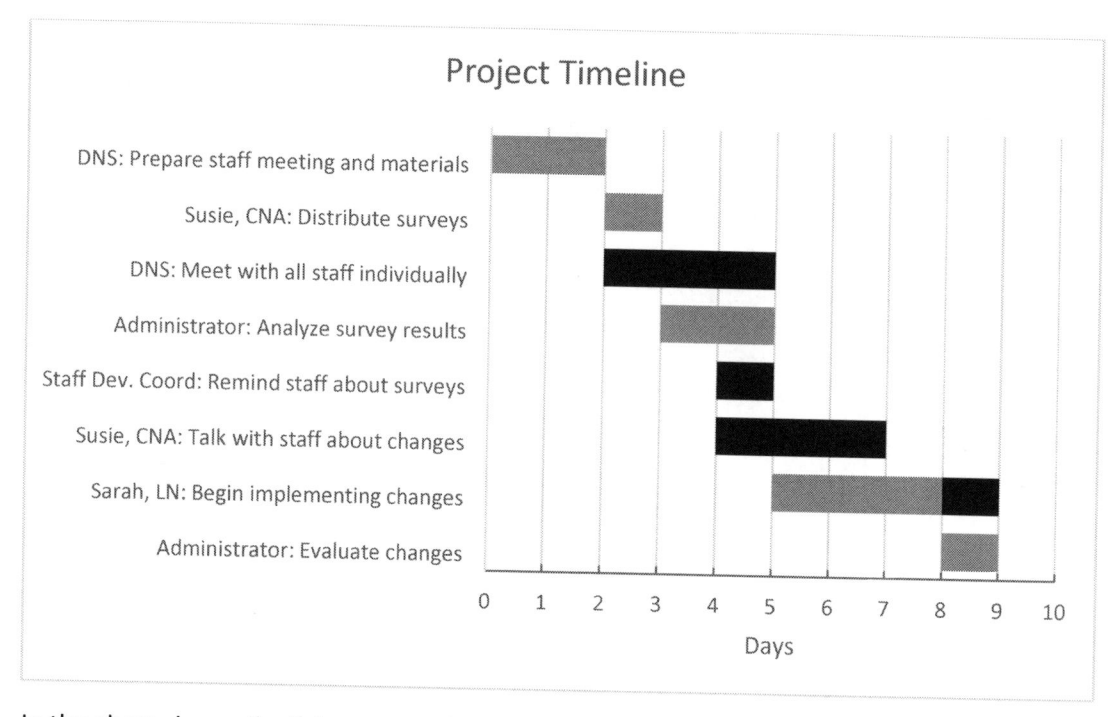

Project Timeline

Task	Days
DNS: Prepare staff meeting and materials	0–2
Susie, CNA: Distribute surveys	2–3
DNS: Meet with all staff individually	2–5
Administrator: Analyze survey results	3–5
Staff Dev. Coord: Remind staff about surveys	4–5
Susie, CNA: Talk with staff about changes	4–7
Sarah, LN: Begin implementing changes	5–9
Administrator: Evaluate changes	8–9

In the chart above, the light areas indicate the critical path of the project: these tasks must be done in a specific sequence. You can't evaluate changes before making the changes! The dark areas are non-critical paths, and other tasks aren't dependent on their completion.

Gantt charts are particularly useful when organizing teams from various departments so that projects don't linger out in space, but instead can be completed as efficiently as possible.

CONTINUOUS IMPROVEMENT AND PROJECT-BASED IMPROVEMENT

Lean is built on the concept of continuous improvement—small improvements made each and every day, along with larger improvements that take time to plan and carry out. Some organizations beginning in their Lean journey hold a "Kaizen Event," or short, intensive improvement session. A Kaizen Event will usually take place over two to five days, with a few weeks of planning beforehand. The team chooses a problem to tackle, conducts extensive root cause analyses, and implements countermeasures and solutions. When the event is completed, the results are displayed and shared for the team to celebrate. Later, Kaizen Events can become regular improvement bursts, designed to keep momentum moving forward.

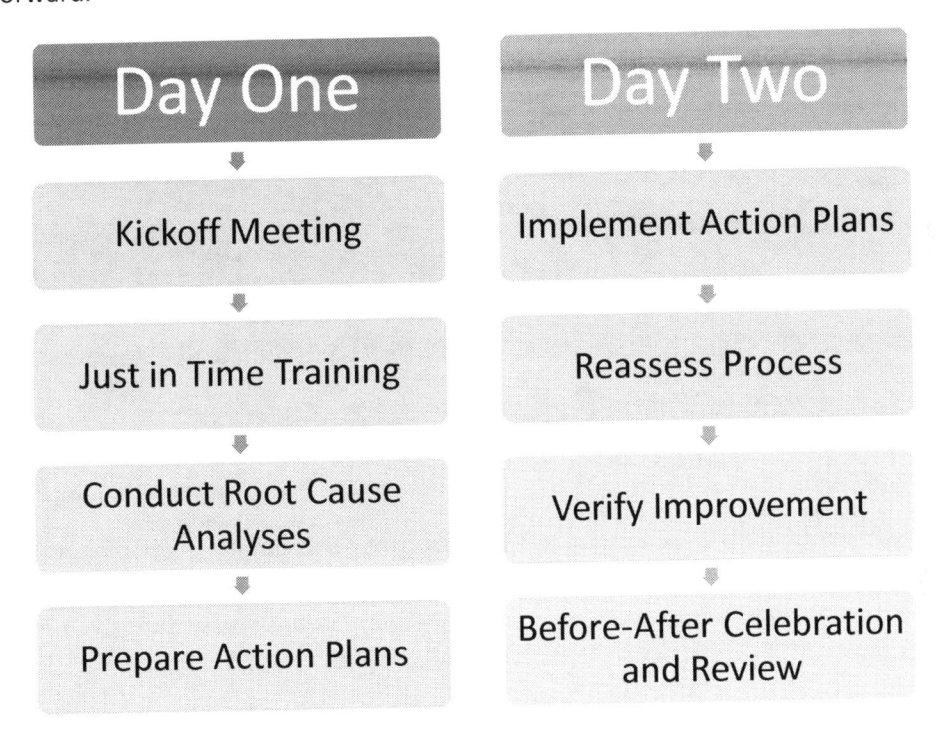

Day One
- Kickoff Meeting
- Just in Time Training
- Conduct Root Cause Analyses
- Prepare Action Plans

Day Two
- Implement Action Plans
- Reassess Process
- Verify Improvement
- Before-After Celebration and Review

For larger projects, A3 templates provide a way to work methodically on a problem. Gathering a team together for an hour or two a week to think deeply about an issue can yield big gains down the line.

An example kaizen event to resolve an issue with supplies of gloves and briefs might look like this:

Day One

Kickoff Meeting
Problem: frequently run out of gloves and briefs in storerooms

⬇

Just in Time Training
5S, PDSA, Check sheets

⬇

Conduct Root Cause Analyses
Talk with line staff; gather data on usage

⬇

Prepare Action Plans
Create 5S Plan and storage guidelines; take pictures of before

Day Two

Implement Action Plans
Apply 5S; display guidelines; remove hoard piles

⬇

Reassess Process
Discuss new guidelines with staff

⬇

Verify Improvement
Watch usage; take pictures of after.

⬇

Before-After Celebration and Review
Create storyboard of work; celebrate with ice cream cones

Kaizen Events work in tandem with building a culture of continuous improvement. Kaizen Events can provide a boost of energy, but they aren't a replacement for providing employees with time every single day to think about improvement opportunities and test interventions.

How can you find the time? At first, it requires a little faith and a small investment. You just have to make the time. Once you start, however, you will quickly find dozens of ways to free up staff time. Don't be tempted to cash out gains early by reducing staff hours or headcount. Invest this time in dedicated improvement work. By building on previous gains, you will magnify your overall investment in Lean many times over.

PROJECT COMPONENTS AND STRUCTURE: A PRIMER

Sponsor: The project sponsor organizes the team, leads the creation of the project charter, and supports the team's activities. Sponsorship of projects is an important aspect of the leadership required to sustain improvement. Project sponsors are individuals who have the authority to make changes in a particular area, who ensure the team stays on track during the project, and who remove barriers and obstacles when necessary. In the beginning, project sponsors are typically department managers.

Should an administrator be a project sponsor? Perhaps, but try to identify another person for each project. When an administrator serves as the project sponsor, particularly at single-site communities, projects are frequently delayed because an administrator is constantly being pulled in different, usually urgent, directions.

Team: Project teams should be between 2 and 10 people, with the ideal number for most projects being 3-6. Teams larger than this typically struggle to meet, organize work, and accomplish goals. Team members should also be willing to work on the project. While it is sometimes useful to involve a naysayer on a project team, be careful to ensure they are committed to the project goal. It is one thing to inspire a reluctant employee who has seen change come and go and quite another to burden a team with someone who will criticize every idea.

Stakeholders: Everyone who will be impacted by the process or improvement is a stakeholder. It's crucial to spend time identifying these groups so engagement and communication plans can be developed and executed. One of the biggest challenges with sustaining change is not properly involving and communicating with stakeholders, which then leads to poor implementation, resentment and pullback.

Charter: A project charter is a document that describes the purpose, the scope (what's included and what's not included) and a shared understanding of what will be accomplished and when. Charters don't need to be fancy; the first box of the A3 document is a good template for most purposes.

Kick-off Meeting: The kick-off meeting is the crucial launch to any project. Here, the team reviews the charter, roles, and expectations, and develops a plan of action including any needed training for the project team. This is also a great time for senior leadership to be present and show support for initiatives, which helps to build awareness and excitement.

Timeline: Make sure the project has a timeline! So many improvement activities in aging services get lost in the daily shuffle, and weeks can turn quickly into months. Establish the timeline in the kick-off meeting after discussion with the project team. It's okay if the timeline is adjusted down the line, but by establishing it upfront, you build momentum to stay on track.

LEADERSHIP AND PROJECT SPONSORSHIP

Strong, involved leadership is crucial to the success of Lean—it's not a program you can implement from your office, or delegate to another staff person. Lean must be led from each level of the organization for it to be successful. Sponsorship is how the project leader accomplishes work through the team. Since projects will be led by a variety of people on the team, it's important to spend time developing the leadership abilities of those project sponsors.

Jim Kouzes and Barry Posner, in <u>The Leadership Challenge</u>, conducted thousands of interviews with successful leaders across industries. They found that leadership isn't a personality or something you are born with; instead, it's an observable set of skills and abilities that can be learned and practiced. They distilled this research into the five practices of exemplary leadership (Kouzes & Posner, 2005):

1. **Practice One—Model the Way**: Leaders set the example for how work should be done and how people should be treated. They remove barriers that inhibit team performance and provide guidance when the path is unclear.

Examples:

- At the end of the day, ask yourself, "What have I done that demonstrated my commitment to the project and team?"
- Work on the floor so that a line staff member can attend training or work on a project
- Be responsive to requests for support and assistance
- Personally check in on project meetings

2. **Practice Two—Inspire a Shared Vision**: Leaders develop a strong idea for what the future will look like, and work hard to communicate that future to others within a framework of goals. Their enthusiasm is contagious and they enlist others in bringing their dreams to reality.

Examples:

- Write out your vision and display it prominently in your office
- Meet with all new employees and share your vision for the work and team
- Discuss improvement projects with residents often, and engage them to share why change is important

3. **Practice Three—Challenge the Process**: Leaders look for ways to change the status quo by improving, improvising and changing how work is done. By experimenting

and taking risks, they discover better ways to accomplish tasks, while gracefully accepting opportunities to learn from mistakes.

Examples:

- Regularly evaluate tasks and meetings and decide if they are still necessary
- Read about innovation occurring in other industries and consider how to apply it to your organization
- Thank people for questioning why work is done a particular way

4. **Practice Four—Enable Others to Act**: Leaders encourage collaboration and increase trust, allowing teams to do more together. By promoting an environment of respect, leaders entrust others with power and capability to join in accomplishing goals.

Examples:

- Meet with team members regularly and find out how you can support them
- Cover floor work so staff can attend training opportunities
- Practice using "we" instead of "I" when describing project work and outcomes to show co-ownership
- Be sure goals and expectations are clear to all

5. **Practice Five—Encourage the Heart**: Leaders spark hope and fire with employees through encouragement and challenge. Leaders celebrate achievements and share rewards of success, thereby creating a strong spirit of community.

Examples:

- Be sure project work and results are displayed prominently to document progress
- Hold a potluck or bake cookies for staff
- Keep a journal for a week or two of all the recognition and rewards you give; evaluate it to make sure you are thanking people adequately
- Invite corporate staff or community leaders to the building to share in team accomplishments

MANAGING CHANGE AND ENCOURAGING INNOVATION

Change is difficult for most people. It usually feels easier and less risky to keep the status quo. People settle into certain procedures and relationships to accomplish work, and, over time, these patterns become expectations and rules for all to follow.

When making changes in organizations, it's important to manage both socio-technical change, that is, the changes of people and work processes, and emotional change, that is, the change process itself as experienced by the people involved. If you are implementing a new dining program, the socio-technical changes would be the menu changes, the different roles of staff, new food items needed, etc. The emotional changes would involve how CNAs feel about serving in the dining, how department managers feel about increased responsibilities, how the foodservice director feels about less oversight over the food program, etc.

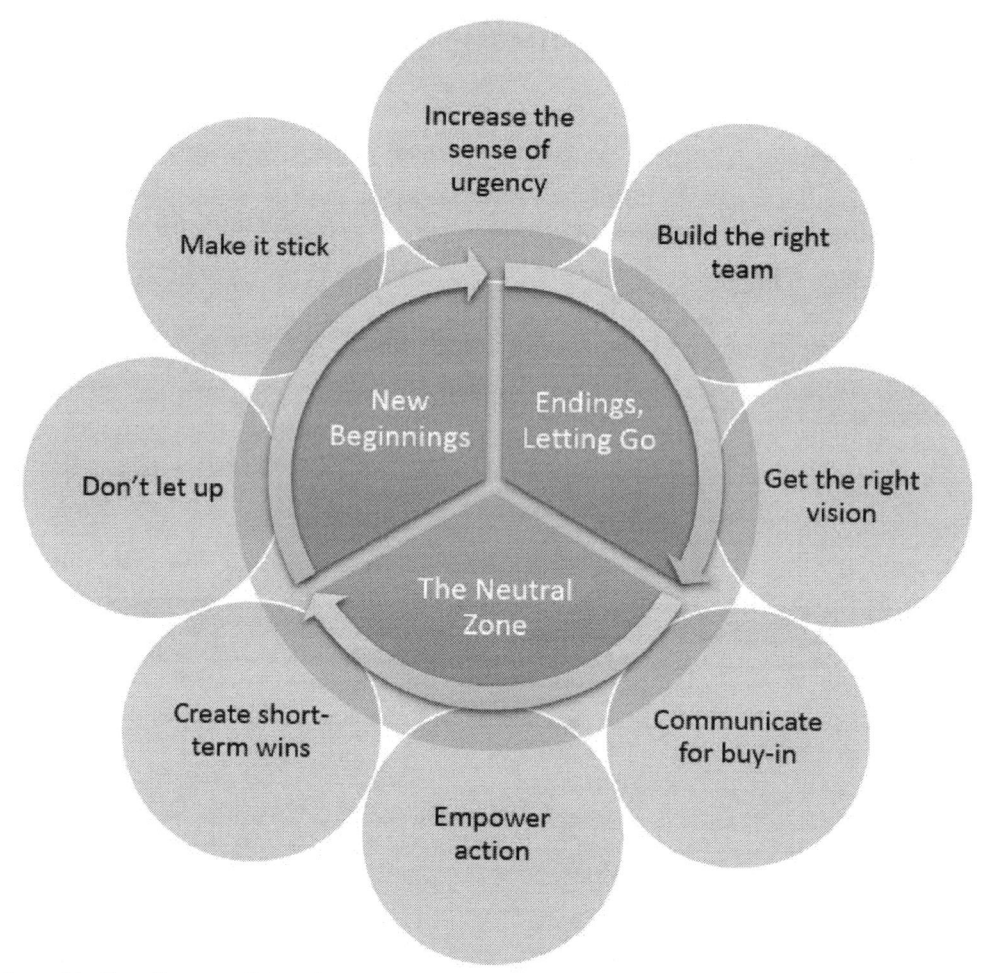

A combination diagram of Kotter's eight points of change with Bridges' three zone model

John Kotter, a well-known leadership professor from Harvard Business School, has studied change initiatives extensively. Specifically, he has looked at why some change efforts succeed while many other change efforts fail. (Kotter estimates that 75% of large organizational change initiatives fail.) Based on his extensive research, Kotter has developed an eight-step model for improving change processes. (Kotter, Leading Change, 2012) The steps are:

1. **Increase the sense of urgency**: People need to understand why they must change. Whether it's a new payment model or different resident expectations, it's important to make the case for change. A common example is to imagine you are on a burning off-shore platform. While jumping into the ocean seems terrifying, it is the only way forward with a chance at survival.
2. **Build the right team**: Once again, the team is crucial to success with changes. Make sure you work hard at building a strong, committed team. In the old days, it may have been important to have staff that followed instructions and didn't rock the boat. Now, however, we need people who can problem solve independently and aren't afraid to speak up when they notice a way to better serve residents.
3. **Get the right vision**: Know where you are trying to go. For most organizations, focusing on the needs of the person served is at the core of their mission, and it's usually fairly easy to align the vision with this mission.
4. **Communicate for buy-in**: Communicate, communicate, and communicate. Use a variety of methods and materials, be frequently present, and engage staff to ensure understanding. Rarely has a change initiative in any organization been over-communicated. Remember that communication is a two-way street, too: don't just shovel out memos and information—listen to feedback and make sure to engage all in the process.
5. **Empower action**: Leaders cannot do everything themselves. Instead, work hard to empower staff to make decisions, and support them, even if the decisions turn out to be wrong. Mistakes are usually the best way to learn how to do better, so take those opportunities to mentor staff rather than punishing them.
6. **Create short-term wins**: Don't begin with a giant, long-term overhaul, as people will tend to lose interest and commitment to progress. Focus on small, visible goals first to build excitement and engagement. One of the reasons why 5S is a great starting place is that it's both easy and plain to see. People see and experience the change and are much more likely to work on larger projects.
7. **Don't let up**: Once a change begins, understand there will be peaks and valleys. Don't give up on the goals and vision. Push forward with focus and dedication to the team.
8. **Make it stick**: For change to be successful long-term, it has to become part of the culture. This is as true for Lean and improvement as anything else. Build improvement thinking into every part of the culture, from orientation to evaluations to celebrations. Ensure that respect for people is practiced by everyone in the

organization and that everyone spends time thoughtfully reflecting on how to do better. (Kotter, Getting Change to Stick, 2011)

William Bridges, in <u>Managing Transitions</u>, developed a model for managing the emotional impact of transitions (Bridges, 2009, pp. 4-5):

1. **Letting go, losing, endings:**

    When implementing change, it's important to recognize the loss associated with letting go of old ways. Oftentimes, the people who struggle the most with this will be the best employees—after all, they have been the most successful in the old system. Spend time preparing for the transition by talking about the reasons for the change and how it will benefit residents. Build up the need for improvement. Also, understand that people are generally more likely to take a risk to minimize a loss (holding on to the status quo, for instance) than to take a risk to obtain a gain (a better process or outcome). That's why even a positive change can be hard for people to accept.

2. **The neutral zone:**

    The neutral zone describes the uncertain area between the old and new. Things are different, but not quite settled. Staff experience confusion and uncertainty in what's happening and where the organization is going. Communicating a strong vision, encouraging people to try even if mistakes occur, and finding short-term goals to mark success are all crucial waypoints to guide the team through the neutral zone.

3. **New beginnings:**

    New beginnings can be exciting, but there is often a tendency to slide back, particularly without active engagement from leaders. At this point, you must work hard to build the new way of working into the very culture of the work area, from training new staff to ensuring that resources and rewards are aligned with the new way.

PRACTICAL STRATEGIES FOR IMPLEMENTING CHANGE

Joel Barker has developed an easy, ten-step model for approaching implementation of innovations and new ideas by addressing certain 'key levers' to make it easier for employees to embrace change initiatives. (Barker, 2008) By studying these levers beforehand, change agents can more effectively craft solutions that will be adopted more easily.

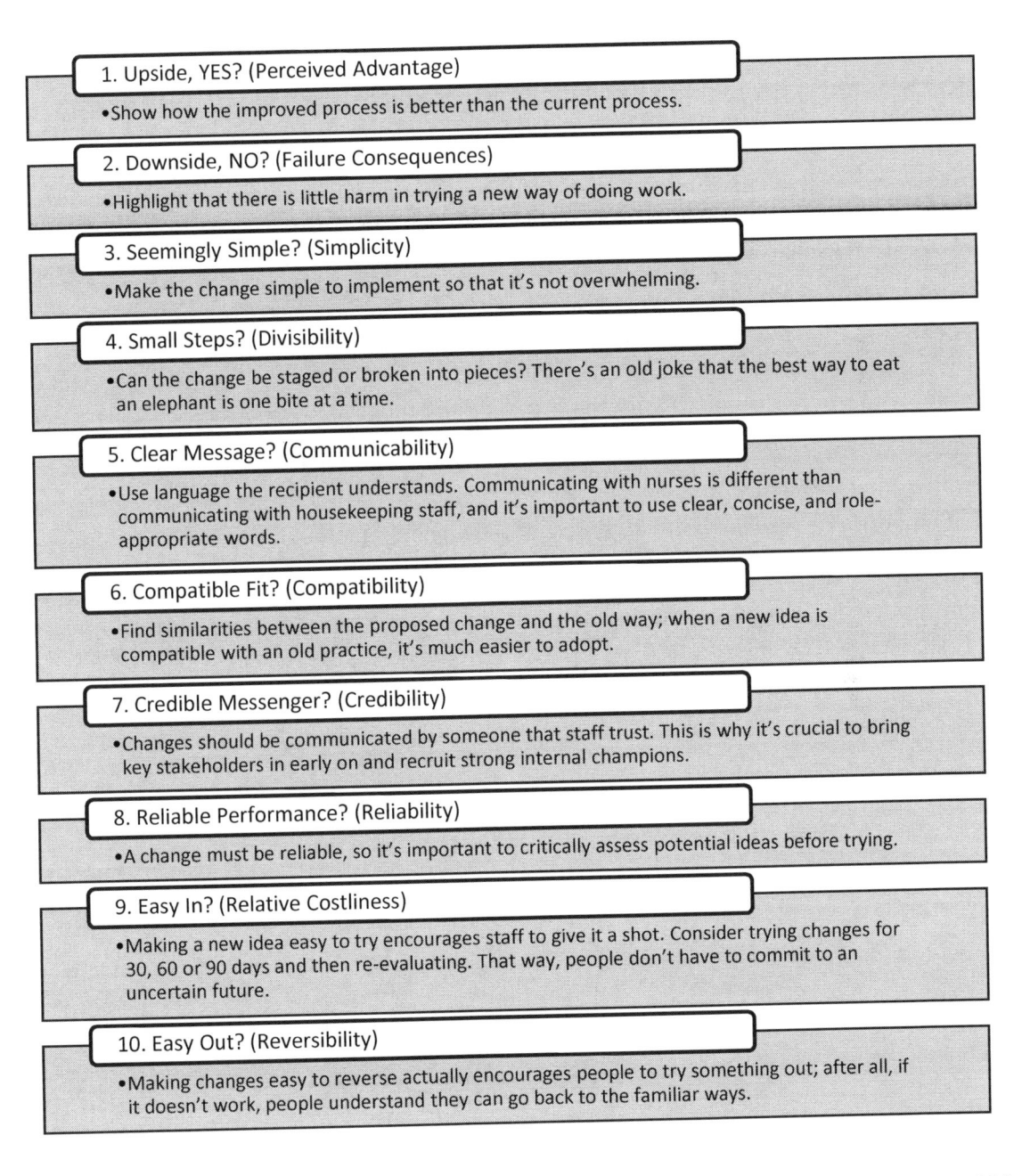

1. Upside, YES? (Perceived Advantage)
- Show how the improved process is better than the current process.

2. Downside, NO? (Failure Consequences)
- Highlight that there is little harm in trying a new way of doing work.

3. Seemingly Simple? (Simplicity)
- Make the change simple to implement so that it's not overwhelming.

4. Small Steps? (Divisibility)
- Can the change be staged or broken into pieces? There's an old joke that the best way to eat an elephant is one bite at a time.

5. Clear Message? (Communicability)
- Use language the recipient understands. Communicating with nurses is different than communicating with housekeeping staff, and it's important to use clear, concise, and role-appropriate words.

6. Compatible Fit? (Compatibility)
- Find similarities between the proposed change and the old way; when a new idea is compatible with an old practice, it's much easier to adopt.

7. Credible Messenger? (Credibility)
- Changes should be communicated by someone that staff trust. This is why it's crucial to bring key stakeholders in early on and recruit strong internal champions.

8. Reliable Performance? (Reliability)
- A change must be reliable, so it's important to critically assess potential ideas before trying.

9. Easy In? (Relative Costliness)
- Making a new idea easy to try encourages staff to give it a shot. Consider trying changes for 30, 60 or 90 days and then re-evaluating. That way, people don't have to commit to an uncertain future.

10. Easy Out? (Reversibility)
- Making changes easy to reverse actually encourages people to try something out; after all, if it doesn't work, people understand they can go back to the familiar ways.

LEADING AND LAGGING INDICATORS AND PROCESS MANAGEMENT

Most organizations collect data of some form on the results of its work. Whether this is clinical outcomes, operational data or financial results, data can be broken into two types of indicators: a leading indicator, or one that will predict performance of a process or outcome, or a lagging indicator, one that describes the past performance of a process or outcome.

Leading and lagging indicators both serve important purposes. Leading indicators help to guide action before negative outcomes occur; they help an organization be proactive. Lagging indicators are useful for monitoring whether a process or outcome is as expected, and can be a useful quality assurance or oversight mechanism.

Most organizations in aging services are very good at collecting lagging indicator data: how many falls occurred last month; facility profit and loss; resident census. Leading indicators are helpful in building sustainable processes, and are worth a closer examination here.

If you are managing the number of falls in your community, the lagging indicator will be the number of falls, or the falls per resident day or some other formulation. A leading indicator will measure risk factors or things that will likely lead to a fall. This might be the number of residents on 9 or more medications, the number of residents on psychotropic medications, the number of residents with a high fall risk assessment, etc.

In the case of resident census, leading indicators might be the number of hospital inquiries or tour requests, the average hospital census, or the number of intent list applicants.

When implementing a Lean program, it's useful to start measuring items like the number of improvement ideas received, the number of improvement projects completed, employee engagement scores, resident satisfaction results, and other related leading indicators of organizational performance. This helps to build a culture of proactive response to challenges, rather than reactive scrambling to fix problems.

TEACHING PDSA: THE MR. POTATO HEAD GAME

PDSA thinking is a crucial skill that develops with experience. For people that have been doing it for some time, PDSA might even seem simple or "obvious common sense." Unfortunately, this perspective can make it difficult to teach other staff who are less familiar with using the improvement process.

Games are a good way to teach PDSA thinking because they are safe, low risk, and (hopefully) a little fun. One such game uses a Mr. Potato Head toy to demonstrate how rapid improvement cycles work.

A Mr. Potato Head toy can be purchased from many retailers for less than $15. To begin the exercise, review the basic concepts of the PDSA cycle. Explain that the primary purpose of the cycle is to choose a problem, identify possible causes and interventions to prevent those causes, test to determine if the interventions are successful, and then further adjustment/ implementation of those interventions, if successful, or a return to the beginning of the process if not.

The goal of the Mr. Potato Head exercise is to discover faster ways to assemble the toy. Begin by asking a volunteer to establish a baseline time. Place all the parts on a table, and explain that the toy must have all of the required parts, i.e. a nose, mouth, ears, arms, etc. Ask the rest of the group to observe the task and think about ways to improve the process in the next cycle. With a stopwatch, record how long it takes the volunteer to assemble the toy. When finished, thank the volunteer and record the time on a board.

Now, ask the group for a few ideas on how to improve the time. Using a group process, narrow the list down to one idea to try. Some examples might be:

- Remove unneeded parts from the table (e.g., only one mouth is needed)
- Place the items on the table in the order that they will be used
- Decide in advance what order to place items onto the toy

Applying only one change, have the volunteer put together the toy again and record the time on the board. Discuss if the change made a difference. If it did, continue the change in the next cycle. If not, have the team think about why the change didn't reduce the time as expected. Apply any learning to the list of ideas to try next.

Repeat the cycle of choosing an idea to test, testing how long it takes to assemble the toy, and determining if the idea helped or not. After five or six cycles, compare the beginning time with the ending time, and discuss how the PDSA process helped to decide how best to assemble the toy. Finally, relate this exercise back to the team's daily work and discuss how the examination, testing, and application process can improve work processes.

PDSA CASE STUDY: ELIMINATING ALARMS FROM SKILLED NURSING CENTER

Since the late 1980's, communities nationwide have taken dramatic steps to reduce the use of physical restraints among their residents. For many, this meant replacing lap belts and limb ties with bed and pull-tab alarms. These alarms attempt to alert staff to a resident about to fall, although studies on their effectiveness are inconclusive, at best. Many professionals now consider alarms to be unneeded, anachronistic, and disruptive to a resident's wellbeing and quality of life—although removing them can be challenging, as Greenville Manor discovered.

When administrators at Greenville first proposed the idea of removing alarms, staff, family members and even some residents worried about the effect on resident safety and security. A small, interdisciplinary team convened to work on the problem. By talking with staff and residents, and conducting online research, the team determined a number of root causes behind resident falls. The team also examined the process by which a nurse added an alarm to a resident's care plan, and noted that very little investigation typically occurred. By organizing fall causes in a Pareto chart, the team was able to target the top 3 reasons and develop an education program to address those causes.

The team developed a test plan to remove an alarm from one resident and measure the results. After two weeks of no increased falls, the test was expanded to include seven additional residents (one nursing section). The team met frequently to analyze fall data and check in with staff involved in the test pilot. During the test, an alarm was discovered on one of the residents. The team quickly investigated and discovered that one of the night shift employees had been absent from a recent team meeting and did not receive the pilot notice in her mailbox. After correcting the issue, the team made a note to follow-up with a night shift focus group to talk about communication challenges and ways to better communicate between shifts.

After one month, the team determined that removing the alarms had actually resulted in a slight decrease in the number of falls in that section. (Later, the team learned that this result was not uncommon in communities that were successful in removing alarms.) The team decided to move forward with expanding the pilot, but to adjust the communication plan to ensure all staff and other stakeholders received adequate notice of the change.

At the next all-staff meeting, the team shared the results of the test, and solicited reactions from other team members. Staff who were involved in the pilot, along with the project team, responded to questions and helped to allay remaining fears about removing alarms throughout the community. Over the next three months, successive neighborhoods removed alarms while staff carefully monitored fall data. A community-wide party celebrated the removal of alarms, and a record of the before and after fall data was prominently displayed in the staff conference room.

PDSA CASE STUDY: REDUCING EMPLOYEE INJURIES

For many aging services providers, employee injuries are a costly reality of the workplace. In addition to workers compensation costs, however, employee injuries can cause scheduling challenges and lower worker morale. Lakeville Management, a small regional provider of assisted living and memory care communities, decided to tackle employee injuries as part of their commitment to deepening their respect towards employees.

To begin, administrators held several small focus groups to solicit information about the current safety culture, the employee injury reporting process, and barriers to implementing changes. With this initial information, the leadership team was able to construct a company-wide survey and identify opportunities to improve their processes.

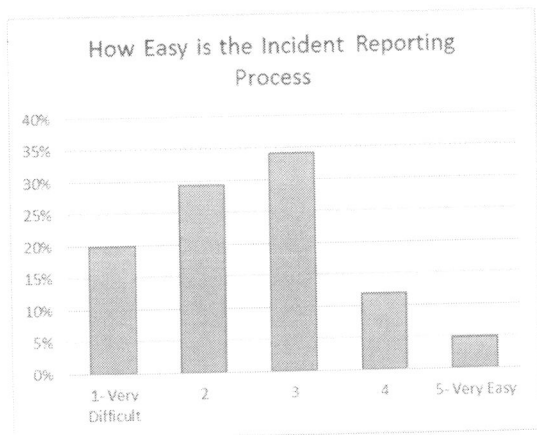

The company safety committee (composed of multi-disciplinary representatives from each member community) first examined their current incident reporting process, which was used to report both actual injuries and near misses. Staff reported that the process was somewhat difficult, and, as a result, very few employees bothered to submit near misses. In addition, by examining the type of injuries that occurred most frequently, the committee decided to focus education and interventions on muscle strains, which accounted for almost 60% of all employee injuries.

The committee began by mapping out the incident reporting process. By dialoguing with supervisors tasked with completing parts of the process, the committee identified pain points, unclear forms, and burdensome back-and-forths. Using this knowledge, the committee tested several process and form updates, refining methods after 30 day trials in a single community.

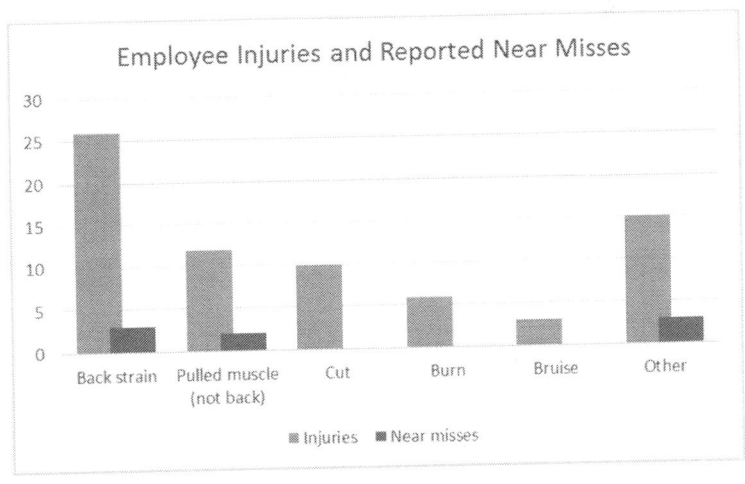

The organization also created a temporary contest to build awareness about the value of near-miss reporting, including incentives for reporting near-misses and a transparent process in each community where near misses and interventions were displayed on a visual control board located in the staff break room. Staff were able see the results of reporting dangers before they led to injuries and could weigh in on interventions to help ensure that proposed changes were realistic within work routines.

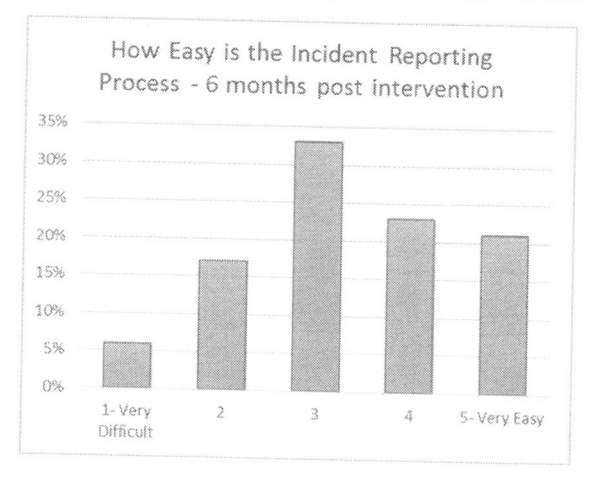

After six months of work and four rounds of the PDSA process, Lakeville reevaluated the incident reporting process ease and short-term results. Supervisors reported that the updated processes were much easier to follow, and the leadership team noted a strong increase in the number of near miss reports. After twelve months, the results were dramatic: almost $200,000 in avoided worker compensation costs, 63% fewer lost days, and 15% fewer modified work days. In addition, managers at Lakeville became accustomed to including a review of staff injuries and near misses as part of their daily work, increasing accountability and awareness for the importance of worker safety to the organization.

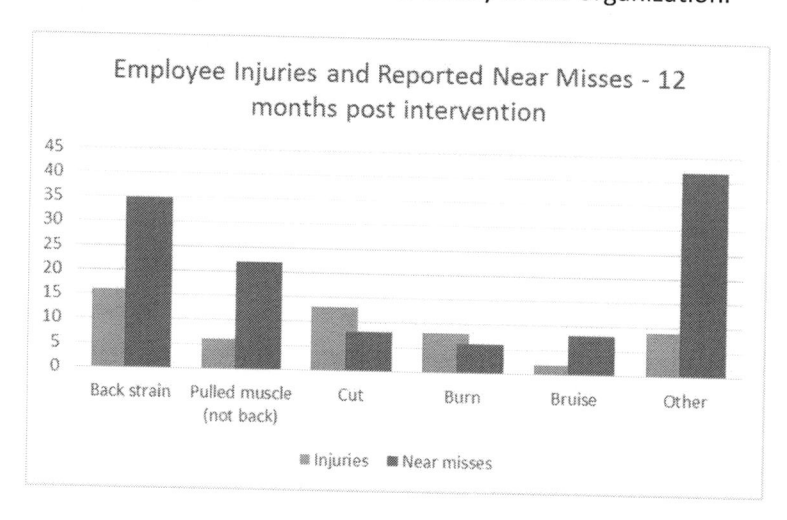

For a similar case study of using lean principles to reduce staff injuries, see "Overcoming Employee Injuries at the Wall" by the Regina Qu'Appelle Health Region: http://www.rqhrlean.com/overcoming-employee-injury-at-the-wall.html

WHAT'S NEXT?

Hopefully by now, you have enough information and tools to begin your Lean journey. Don't worry if you stumble along the way—Toyota still stumbles, and they've been doing it for over 50 years. The key to success is developing an organization that thrives around the concept of continuous improvement; that every day, each member of the organization looks at how he or she can improve the daily work, that each department looks at how it can serve residents better, and that the organization itself looks at how it can build capacity within each member of its team.

There are a tremendous number of books and online resources for each part of the journey. Some are specific to philosophy (e.g. building culture, deepening respect), some to methodology (e.g. daily standard work, A3 thinking, value stream mapping), and some to tools (e.g., 5S, root cause analysis, process maps). Remember that each component is important: applying Lean tools without developing a culture that respects each person will not be sustainable; adopting a Lean philosophy without developing problem solving skills will produce a willing, but unfocused workforce.

Aging services organizations also need to share their experiences, struggles and successes implementing Lean with other providers. Reach out to colleagues to offer advice and seek support. Talk with your hospital partners about their Lean efforts and ask for help with improving inter-system processes. Encourage your provider associations to develop Lean-specific training opportunities and forums. Join Lean healthcare networks[1] and share in the growing resources provided by large hospitals and health systems. Together, we can improve the experience for all of those we serve.

---

[1] The Healthcare Value Network is currently the largest network of healthcare organizations working on Lean improvement. Find out more at their website: http://createvalue.org/networks/healthcare-value-network/

RECOMMENDED LIBRARY FOR FURTHER READING

Lean Hospitals: Improving Quality, Patient Safety and Employee Engagement by Mark Graban

The Toyota Way: 14 Management Principles from the World's Greatest Manufacturer by Jeffrey Liker

Transforming Health Care: Virginia Mason Medical Center's Pursuit of the Perfect Patient Experience by Charles Kenney

Healthcare Kaizen: Engaging Front-Line Staff in Sustainable Continuous Improvements by Mark Graban

Beyond Heroes: A Lean Management System for Healthcare by Kim Barnas

Empowered Work Teams for Long-Term Care by Dale Yeatts, Cynthia Cready and Linda Noelker

On the Mend: Revolutionizing Healthcare to Save Lives and Transform the Industry by John Toussaint

Lean Thinking: Banish Waste and Create Wealth in Your Corporation by James Womack

Regina Qu'Appelle Health Region Lean Website: http://www.rqhrlean.com/

Toyota Kata by Mark Rother

The Lean Glossary: http://www.gembutsu.com/articles/leanmanufacturingglossary.html

BIBLIOGRAPHY

Agency for Healthcare Research and Quality. (n.d.). *Curriculum Tools*. Retrieved 06 13, 2014, from AHRQ: http://www.ahrq.gov/professionals/education/curriculum-tools/index.html

Akao, Y. (2004). *Hoshin Kanri: Policy Deployment for Successful TQM*. New York: Productivity Press.

Anderson, R. A., Issel, L. M., & McDaniel, R. R. (2003). Nursing Homes as Complex Adaptive Systems: Relationship Between Management Practice and Resident Outcomes. *Nursing Research*, 12-21.

Balle, M. (2014, 07 28). *Lead With Respect*. Retrieved from Lean Enterprise Institute: http://www.lean.org/Search/Documents/159.pdf

Barker, J. (2008). *Tactics of Innovation*. Saint Paul: Star Thrower Distribution.

Bridges, W. (2009). *Managing Transitions: Making the Most of Change* (3rd ed.). Philadelphia: De Capo Press.

Deming, W. E. (2000). *Out of the Crisis* (Rev. ed.). Cambridge: MIT Press.

Eden Alternative. (n.d.). *Warmth Surveys*. Retrieved 09 10, 2014, from Eden Alternative: http://www.edenalt.org/resources/warmth-surveys/

Galsworth, G. (2005). *Visual Workplace/ Visual Thinking: Creating Enterprise Excellence Through the Technologies of the Visual Workplace*. Portland: Visual Lean Enterprise Press.

Graban, M. (2011, December 20). *Will Suggestion Boxes be a Trend in 2012? What Method(s) do we Need for Employee Engagement?* Retrieved from LeanBlog: http://www.leanblog.org/2011/12/will-suggestion-boxes-be-a-trend-in-2012-what-methods-for-employee-engagement/

Graban, M. (2012). *Lean Hospitals* (2nd ed.). Boca Raton: CRC Press.

Improvement, I. f. (2014, 09 22). *How to Improve*. Retrieved 09 22, 2014, from Institute for Healthcare Improvement: http://www.ihi.org/resources/Pages/HowtoImprove/default.aspx

Jimmerman, C. (2007). *A3 Problem Solving for Healthcare*. Boca Raton: CRC Press.

Kayyali, A. (2014 Sep). The Impact of Turnover in Nursing Homes. *Am J Nurs*, 69-70.

Kotter, J. (2011, 10 05). *Getting Change to Stick*. Retrieved from Forbes: http://www.forbes.com/sites/johnkotter/2011/10/05/getting-change-to-stick/

Kotter, J. (2012). *Leading Change.* Boston: Harvard Business Review Press.

Kouzes, J., & Posner, B. (2005). *The Leadership Challenge.* New York: Wiley.

Liker, J. (2004). *The Toyota Way: 14 Management Principles from the World's Greatest Manufacturer.* New York: McGraw-Hill.

Meadows, S., Baker, K., & Butler, J. (2014, 08 10). *The Incident Decision Tree: Guidelines for Action following Patient Safety Incidents.* Retrieved from AHRQ: http://www.ahrq.gov/professionals/quality-patient-safety/patient-safety-resources/resources/advances-in-patient-safety/index.html

Mukamel, D. B., Spector, W. D., Limcangco, R., & et al. (2009). The costs of turnover in nursing homes. *Medical Care*, 1039-1045.

Ohno, T. (1988). *Toyota Production System: Beyond Large Scale Production.* New York: Productivity Press.

Petrovich, H. (2015, 06 11). *Study: LTC nurses spend less than half of time on resident care.* Retrieved from McKnight's Long Term Care News: http://www.mcknights.com/news/study-ltc-nurses-spend-less-than-half-of-time-on-resident-care/article/420253/

Protzman, C., Mayzell, G., & Kerpchar, J. (2011). *Leveraging Lean in Healthcare.* New York: Productivity Press.

Rosenthal, M. (2002). *The Essence of Jidoka.* Retrieved from Lean Thinker: http://theleanthinker.com/wp-content/uploads/2009/04/The-Essence-of-Jidoka-SME-Version.pdf

Schroeder, D. M., & Robinson, A. G. (2014). *The Idea Driven Organization.* San Francisco: Berret-Koehler Publishers.

Shook, J. (2011, 6 21). *How to Go to the Gemba: Go See, Ask Why, Show Respect.* Retrieved 7 15, 2014, from Lean Enterprise Institute: http://www.lean.org/shook/displayobject.cfm?o=1843

Smith, M., & Erwin, J. (n.d.). *Role & Responsibility Charting: RACI.* Retrieved from Project Management Institute California Inland Empire Chapter: https://pmicie.org/images/downloads/raci_r_web3_1.pdf

Taylor, M., McNicolas, C., Nicolay, C., & Darzi, A. (2013). Systematic review of the application of the plan–do–study–act method to improve quality in healthcare. *BMJ Quality & Safety.* Retrieved from http://qualitysafety.bmj.com/content/early/2013/09/11/bmjqs-2013-001862.full

The WD-40 Company. (n.d.). *History of the WD-40 Company*. Retrieved 8 14, 2014, from The WD-40 Company: http://www.wd40company.com/about/history/

Womack, J. (1990). *The Machine That Changed the World.* New York: Rawson Associates Scribner.

ABOUT THE AUTHOR

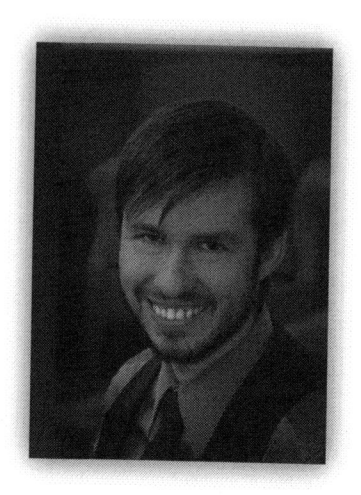

Sean Carey is a licensed nursing home administrator, consultant and frequent speaker on implementing Lean in aging services. After an unrewarding career in hospitality, he serendipitously found work in a small, rural nursing home where he cooked breakfast and laughed with residents. Hooked on the experience, he's spent the last ten years working with aging services providers in skilled nursing, assisted living, senior housing and continuing care retirement communities.

Sean is currently a principal with eSSee Consulting, providing quality improvement, process assessment, Lean training, and technology integration services. A lifelong believer in empowering people to live the life they want, Sean believes that Lean, at its core, is a project of democratic engagement of human potential. He is committed to helping organizations better serve residents, staff, and stakeholders by improving quality, reducing waste, and building long-term value.

You may contact Sean by email at sean@essee.us or by visiting his website: http://www.seancarey.me.

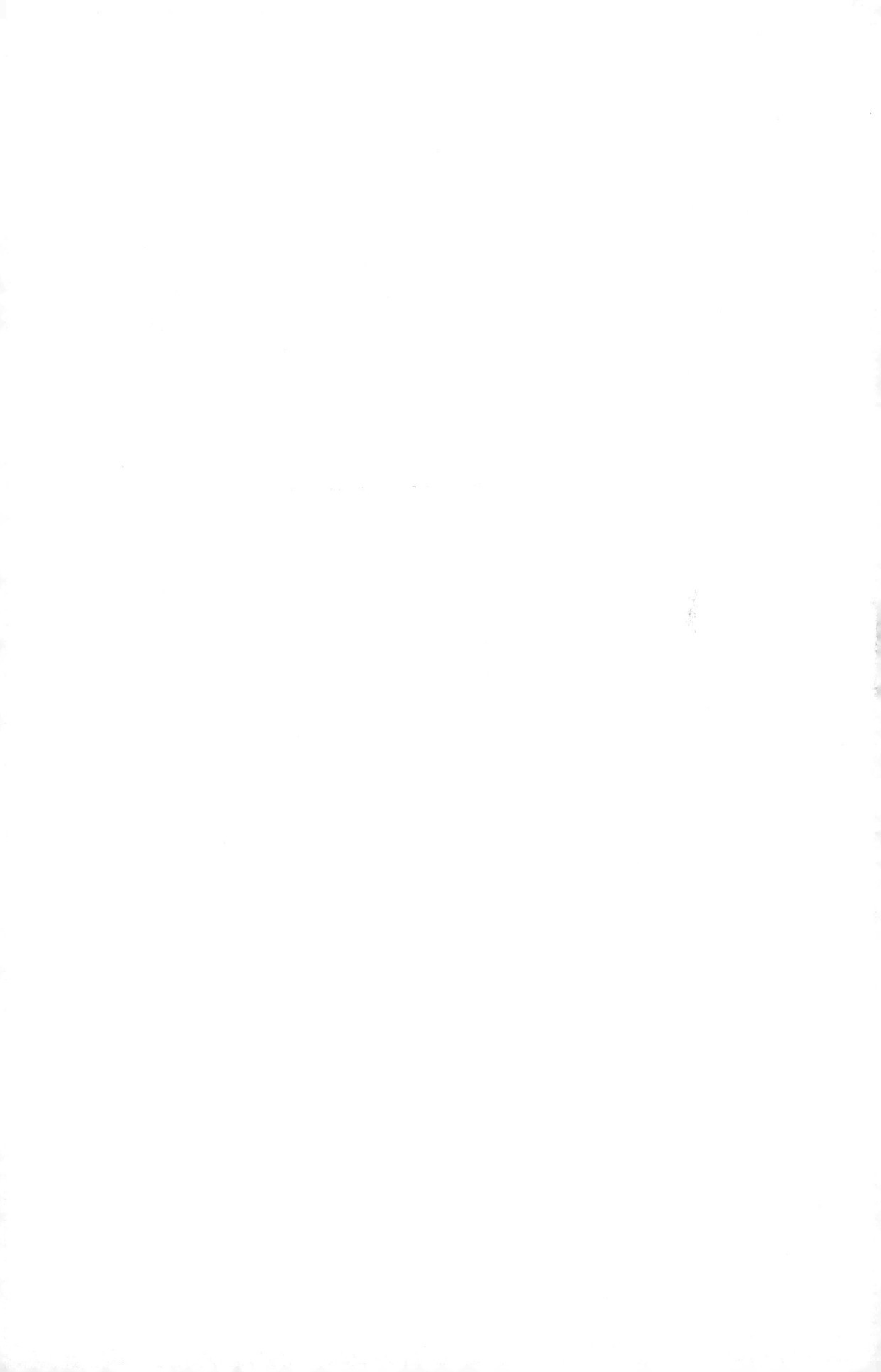

Made in the USA
Middletown, DE
11 January 2018